Tinnitus:
The Complete Self-Help Guide

Revised and Updated by
Julia Clerk

Original Work by
Bill Habets

United Research Publishers

Published in the United States by United Research Publishers as *Tinnitus: The Complete Self-Help Guide.*

ISBN 1-887053-20-4

Published in 2000/2002 by United Research Publishers as *The Tinnitus Handbook, A Self Help Guide.*
Published in Great Britain by Carnell plc as *The Complete Guide to Tinnitus.*

Book and cover design by The Art Deptartment, Green Valley, AZ.

Order additional copies from:

United Research Publishers
P.O. Box 232344
Encinitas, CA 92023-2344
Phone: 760-930-8937

To view our complete range of titles or to order on-line, visit our web site: **www.urpublishers.com**

Contents

13 Where to Get More Information— International Resources   191

Foreword

Tinnitus is a very common disorder that affects an estimated one in four American adults. Despite this high prevalence, relatively few studies are currently being funded into finding out how tinnitus can be alleviated. Nevertheless, research continues. While no one is predicting any dramatic breakthrough soon, there is a steady accumulation of greater understanding of what causes tinnitus, how it may be prevented, and - perhaps most importantly - how its symptoms can be alleviated by a wide range of therapies.

In the meantime, after running through the whole gamut of what professionals can offer, many a tinnitus sufferer is eventually faced with the conclusion that his or her condition hasn't been cured and essentially remains unchanged. This doesn't mean there isn't a great deal that can be done to minimize both the symptoms and impact of tinnitus. It just means that help will not necessarily come from traditional medical sources. As many sufferers will testify, planning and executing your own self-help program is often an excellent way to bring tinnitus under control. Naturally, it's important that before you embark on such a course, you should undertake all of the medical tests necessary to exclude the possibility that your tinnitus is caused by some other underlying disorder that can be cured by medical intervention.

Because self-help is so often the key to making tinnitus fade into lesser significance, a large part of this book is devoted to providing recommendations and suggestions for self-help techniques. However, as you read on, please bear two most important points in mind.

Firstly, a book like this cannot be - nor is it intended to be - in any way a substitute for professional medical advice. Readers are urged to consult their doctor before trying any therapy not prescribed by medically-qualified professionals. Only your own doctor can help you decide what may or may not be helpful or appropriate in the specific circumstances of your own case.

Secondly, although the information offered in this book is based upon the views of doctors, specialists and other health professionals, these experts are by no means always in agreement on many aspects of tinnitus. In many cases, there are dissenting opinions. Whenever this is the case, we have tried to provide a balanced view of all sides of a particular argument.

Finally, we would like to say "thank you" to all those who have given so generously of their time and expertise during our research. While they are too many to mention individually, to each and every one of them, our sincere and appreciative thanks.

CHAPTER 1

What is Tinnitus?

Tinnitus has been defined by the American Tinnitus Association (ATA) as the "perception of sound in one or both ears or in the head when no external sound is present." The word "tinnitus" comes from the Latin word *tinnere* which means "to ring like a bell." Maybe that explains why tinnitus is so often described as a ringing in the ears. However, tinnitus sufferers can experience a range of sounds—from whistling and chirping to clicking, roaring or hissing. The ATA explains that tinnitus can be intermittent or constant—with single or multiple tones—and its perceived volume can range from subtle to shattering.

Tinnitus has two pronunciations: ti-NIGHT-us or TIN-i-tus. While both forms are correct, the ATA tends to use the former. Within the mainstream medical community there is some confusion about whether tinnitus is a disorder in its own right or merely a label that conveniently identifies a number of broadly similar symptoms.

The National Institute on Deafness and Other Communication Disorders (NIDCD) says that tinnitus is a symptom associated with many forms of hearing loss and can also be a symptom of other health problems.

Craniosacral therapist Julian Cowan Hill, R.C.S.T., on the other hand, declares that tinnitus is a state in which the ears have become too sensitive and this hypersensitive listening detects the noises of the brain. Adding to the ambiguity surrounding tinnitus is a famous 1953 experiment by Heller and Bergman in which it was found that the vast majority of people with "normal" hearing (93% of their sample) heard buzzing, pulsing or whistling sounds in their head or ears when immersed in total silence.

In a nutshell, experts agree that tinnitus is usually caused by (or amplified by) one of the following:

◊   Hearing loss of different types

◊   Wax build-up in the ear canal

◊   Ear or sinus infections

⬧ Exposure to loud noise (on a one-off basis or over prolonged periods of time)

⬧ Head or neck trauma

⬧ Prolonged use of one or more of over 200 types of medicine (ototoxic drugs)

⬧ Other health problems including circulatory system ailments, diabetes, allergies and (very rarely) tumors

A Very Ancient Problem

Because many forms of tinnitus are the result of over-exposure to very loud noise levels over lengthy periods of time, it is assumed by some people that the complaint is a malady of modern times and perhaps didn't exist when life was simpler and probably less noisy. It's a nice theory, but one that's not borne out by the facts. References to tinnitus can be found in the earliest medical writings, dating back to the dawn of civilization in Mesopotamia and Egypt.

It's difficult to determine whether or not tinnitus is actually on the increase, although there is plenty of evidence to suggest that there are now more recorded cases than ever before. Of course, this leaves open the question as to how tinnitus was diagnosed in the past. Many cases might have gone unrecorded. Most experts agree, however, that it's very likely that more people have tinnitus today—or are at greater risk of eventually developing it—than ever before. Factors that may have contributed to this rise include:

- ◊ Many cases of tinnitus can be traced back to previous exposure to sounds that were loud enough to cause hearing loss. Modern technology has brought us an endless variety of home entertainment in the form of television, music systems and DVD players as well as portable audio and video devices which we can listen to for long periods of time at volumes high enough to ultimately damage hearing.

- ◊ There is little doubt that our towns and cities have generally become noisier places, with the cumulative effect of this noise pollution taking a toll on the hearing of the inhabitants. There is also some evidence to suggest that tinnitus stemming from working or having previously worked in noisy environments may be on the increase despite various government regulations meant to control noise levels in the workplace.

- ◊ Even medical advances in other fields may contribute to the increasing the risk of tinnitus. Several drugs used to treat quite ordinary conditions have been

found to trigger the problem in susceptible people.

◊   A very common form of tinnitus is the one
that is associated with hearing loss that
occurs mainly as part of the aging process.
As more people live longer, greater num-
bers reach the age when tinnitus is likely
to become noticeable.

Incidence and Prevalence

When considering how widespread tinnitus is,
there are two separate aspects to take into account: its prevalence and incidence:

◊   **Prevalence:** A measurement based on
the number of people affected by the condition in a given population (also called
prevalence rate).

◊   **Incidence:** A measurement of the number
of new episodes of an illness or disorder arising in a given population over a specific period of time. Incidence is most often expressed as the number of episodes of the disorder per 1,000 individuals at risk (also called
the *incidence rate* or *inception rate*).

While there is agreement amongst experts that
tinnitus is extremely common, there is some dis-

crepancy between statistics from various sources which may all boil down to definitions.

The American Tinnitus Association estimates that over 50 million Americans suffer from tinnitus to some degree, with about 12 million of these people having it severe enough to seek medical attention. Two million of these people are so seriously affected that they cannot hear, work or sleep normally. The Mayo Clinic, on the other hand, estimates that some 36 million Americans have tinnitus to a "distressing degree."

Experts generally agree that tinnitus affects males and females in equal ratios and is most common between the ages of 40 and 70. However, it can sometimes affect children. While statistics are undoubtedly open to interpretation or liable to slight error, there is little doubt that tinnitus is a health problem of massive proportions, affecting perhaps as much as a quarter of the population at one time or another.

If your tinnitus is caused by another health problem (e.g. like wax build-up in the ear), your doctor may well be able to treat the condition and lessen the noise. But if your tinnitus is due to age-related hearing loss or damage to the ears due to exposure to excessive noise, medical practitioners often offer little hope. In fact, the NIDCD declares quite frankly that "there is no cure for tinnitus."

However, this viewpoint may be bleaker than the reality. Most tinnitus sufferers don't have to face a torturous future. Hundreds of thousands of sufferers—some of them with very severe tinnitus—have found ways of overcoming or minimizing their problem using methods and techniques like those described in later chapters.

CHAPTER 2

Normal Hearing & Sound Perception

Before turning our attention to how tinnitus interferes with hearing, it's useful to consider what sounds someone with "normal" hearing should be able to recognize and differentiate.

The three main fundamental characteristics of any given sound are its pitch, loudness and timbre. The ability to clearly hear each of these constituent components varies greatly, even in people considered to have normal hearing. Let us look at each of these components in turn:

Pitch

The pitch of a sound is how quickly or slowly the object producing that sound vibrates—the faster the vibration, the higher the pitch of that sound will be. Generally, the shorter or smaller the vibrating object, the higher will be the pitch of the sounds it produces.

For example, the strings producing the high notes found at the extreme right end of an acoustic piano's keyboard are much shorter than those producing the deep bass notes triggered by keys at the extreme left of the keyboard. Equally, notes available on a trumpet—which is comparatively small% fall in a much higher range than those you can get from a tuba, a much larger instrument. (Naturally, in these days of synthesized sounds, the size of an electronic instrument no longer indicates whether it will be high- or low-pitched.)

Pitch is measured by how many times the sound-producing source vibrates in one second. This measurement is called cycles per second (cps) but is also frequently expressed as "hertz" (a term often abbreviated to Hz). One Hz represents one cycle per second; 10,000 Hz means that the vibrations repeat 10,000 times every second. A thousand Hz is also often shown as one kHz (one kilohertz).

Normally, humans can hear sounds occurring within the range of about 15 cycles per second to 20,000 cycles. However, it's common for the upper limit to substantially reduce as you get older, the upper audibility mark falling to perhaps as little as half of what you might have had when you were younger. The human ear can usually detect sounds lower than 15 cycles per second, but what's actually discerned is an ill-defined rumble lacking any definite pitch and which may be felt or sensed rather than heard. Sounds above 20,000 cycles are, however, totally inaudible to the vast majority of adults. Children can often hear sounds pitched as high as 40,000 cycles, but this ability begins to tail off by around 1000 cycles per year once maturity has been reached.

Loudness

While the loudness of a sound is determined by the amount of energy it releases—banging a drum with great force will create a louder sound than tapping it lightly—the way in which loudness is perceived by the human ear is also affected by the pitch of the sound. Not all pitches are equal as far as the human ear is concerned. It will hear some more clearly (and therefore more loudly) than others.

⬥ Hearing is most sensitive to sounds falling in what's called the "middle high tones range" which encompasses frequencies from about 1,000 to about 4,000 cycles per second. A person's ability to hear sounds in these frequencies is so developed that, were it any greater, we would begin to audibly discern the movement of air particles.

⋄ Hearing sensitivity drops off gradually below about 1,000 cycles. It's just as well that we cannot hear sounds below a certain pitch because otherwise, we would be under constant attack from low frequency sounds produced within our own body, like those resulting from bone and muscle movements.

⋄ Hearing sensitivity reduces sharply above the 4,000-cycle ceiling, and does so much more rapidly than the drop-off at the lower level. Incidentally, stereos and many television sets have a "loudness control" that you can switch on when listening at low volume in order to deliberately counteract the ear's greater sensitivity to middle tones. This control boosts the relative volume of sounds both in the lower bass and upper treble regions, restoring the overall *perceived* balance to more or less that which you would hear with the control switched off and the main volume turned up higher.

To put these ranges in perspective, the fundamental of the musical note middle C or *do* (located just to the left of the keyboard's centre) played on a correctly-tuned piano will vibrate at

256 cycles. As the number of vibrations doubles or halves an octave higher or lower, a standard piano's highest note (the top C at the extreme right) vibrates at more than 4,000 times a second and the instrument's lowest note (the A at the extreme left) vibrates 27.5 times a second, or nearly twice as fast as the average low-pitch audibility threshold.

However, many sounds don't have a definite pitch like that produced by musical instruments and are instead a combination of many different pitches so interwoven that no single specific pitch can be discerned. Sounds without specific pitch are known as "noises." The term takes on a somewhat different meaning in this context. Typical examples of noise might include sounds like those made by boiling water or the clatter of horse hooves. Naturally, when the sound is a noise, the ear's sensitivity to pitch plays little role in determining how loudly it is heard.

The range of loudness to which a healthy ear can respond is vast, the ratio having been calculated as a hundred million to one, meaning that the loudest recognizable sound may be a hundred thousand thousand times louder than the faintest one which can still be heard.

Loudness is expressed in decibels (abbreviated as dB), a unit for indicating the relative intensity of sounds. The decibel level derives from a logarithmic calculation applied to a measurement of the variation that a given sound source creates in the sound pressure of the air molecules. However, because the human ear has varying sensitivity to different ranges of pitches, the standard decibel measurement is usually converted to a different form that takes this into account, known as dB(A).

This unit of measurement is used most often to express loudness levels as they relate to human hearing. To put this into perspective, here are the approximate dB(A) levels for some common sounds, based upon the assumption that the listener is comparatively near their source:

⬦ Only just audible ambient sounds, such as those you might hear on a still day if you really listened for them—10dB(A).

⬦ Whispered conversation—40 dB(A).

⬦ Normal conversation—60 dB(A).

⬦ Shouting loudly—80 dB(A).

⬦ Symphony orchestra during a loud passage—100 dB(A).

⬦ Jet airplane at full thrust (during take-off)—in excess of 120 dB(A).

⬦ Sound level peaks at a rock concert—130-140 dB(A)

◊ Firing of medium-caliber rifle—160 dB(A).

Just where the thresholds of painful and/or harmful noise lie varies somewhat from person to person. Different experts also have conflicting views on this, but the following will serve as a point of reference:

◊ It's generally agreed that damage to hearing may result following prolonged exposure to sounds in excess of 90 decibels.

◊ Sounds in excess of 130 decibels are likely to be physically painful to endure and will likely cause damage.

The loudness of a sound is also related to the distance separating the listener from its source. In fact, scientists differentiate sharply between the intensity of a sound (this being a measurable physical quantity) and its loudness (this being the product of both the sound's intensity and how sensitive the ear is to it under the currently prevailing conditions).

Because our perception of loudness is also affected by our reaction to the kind of sound we're hearing, it can be difficult to state at exactly what level sound becomes obtrusive. For example, if you love Wagner, you may well find the crescendo in *Ride of the Valkyries* totally acceptable at 100 decibels. However, should the same relative level of loudness be produced by your neighbor's children playing the latest rap music, then you may well think of this as being excruciatingly painful.

Two other factors that affect just how "loudly" we hear something:

1. The human brain generally does an excellent job in filtering out what we want to hear from sounds of little or no interest to us. For example, parents often hear *their* child's voice more clearly than those of the other children when they're all singing at more or less the same volume in a choir.

2. When there are many sounds of varying volumes, the one with the consistently highest pitch will usually be heard most sharply, even though its volume many be lower than that of many of the other sounds. This phenomenon explains why—apart from what sound engineers may have done with relative volumes when mixing a recording—a singer's voice (normally treble) soars distinctively above the accompaniment (normally in the bass or middle regions).

Timbre

The third major component by which a sound is identified is timbre, that quality which makes a particular sound what it is. For example, why a piano sounds like a piano and not a trumpet.

Virtually all sounds incorporate a number of what might be called "sub-sounds," except that these additional sounds are pitched higher than the one we hear most clearly. For example, if you strike middle C on a piano, the string struck by the hammer will vibrate at 256 cycles per second. However, apart from vibrating along its whole length, the string also vibrates in halves—the two halves, of course, being exactly half the length of the whole string. These two halves will vibrate exactly twice as fast, producing a fainter but still discernible note sounding exactly an octave higher than the one being played (the fundamental). The creation of overtones doesn't stop at just halves because the piano's string also vibrates in thirds, quarters and so on, each of these subdivisions of the string producing sounds that are pitched higher, until they are so high that they can no longer be heard by the human ear.

The sounds produced by the vibrations of only a part of the string are called overtones, harmonics or partials and it's the relative volume of these that gives an instrument its peculiar and distinctive sound. For example, a good piano will produce quite strong overtones throughout the audible range, while a clarinet will produce almost no overtones. Because, by definition, overtones are pitched higher than their fundamental, it's quite common for some of these to fall into a range beyond that which humans can hear, especially when our upper hearing range has become restricted. When that happens, we may have difficulty in fully interpreting or understanding the source sound because we fail to capture enough of its overtones.

Another distinguishing mark of any sound is the *attack envelope,* a phrase that describes the manner in which that sound first manifests itself and then continues. Broadly speaking, there are two main types of attacks:

1. *Percussive sounds* are those which start off loudly and whose loudness then reduces rapidly. The piano and guitar are two common examples of instruments producing percussive sounds. Typical examples of nonmusical percussive sounds include thunderclaps or the snap of a twig.

2. *Constant sounds* are those that alter little while being produced, like those coming from a flute or a church organ.

There is also a third form of attack, one in which the sound starts off at low volume, then gradually becomes louder and louder. Incidentally, many sounds incorporate more than one form of attack, with some aspects of the sound gradually rising in volume while others remain constant or diminish.

Human speech, according to what is being said and how it is being said, can be either mainly percussive or mainly constant, depending upon whether the speaker adopts a staccato or sing-song delivery. The manner of speech—apart from whether the speaker has a high- or low-pitched voice and speaks loudly or softly—clearly influences the extent to which it may be heard clearly by someone whose hearing is less than perfect.

Sound Transmission

Of particular relevance to some forms of tinnitus is how sound is transmitted. Generally speaking, the medium of transmission is the air, which responds to the vibrations created by the object making the sound picked up by the human ear. However, solids can also act as excellent sound transmitters. One obvious example is the "listening sticks" used by water company inspectors to detect leaks in underground pipes.

Similarly, the human ear may hear sounds which are brought to it via the bones or the tissues of the body.

Liquids, too, are good sound transmitters, as evidenced by how electronic devices can track submarines many miles away. Equally, the liquids in the body (like blood) can act as a conduit bringing sound sensations to the ear.

Summing Things Up

All sounds—and therefore all noises—consist of a number of different components, some of which may be more or less audible to a given individual, according to the state of his or her hearing. In the next chapter, we will look at the sounds associated with tinnitus, many of which have no obvious source.

CHAPTER 3

The Sounds of Tinnitus

While tinnitus is generally defined as "noises heard in the ear in the absence of matching noises in the surrounding environment," this definition fails to point out that tinnitus can also result from hearing sounds that exist within the body itself rather than in the surrounding environment.

There are many forms of tinnitus. And experts have created a wide variety of labels to define its various subdivisions. But essentially the disorder can be broadly classified into one of the following four main categories:

1.   *Objective tinnitus* occurs when the noises that you hear are real enough, although of a kind that most people don't normally hear. In such instances, the sounds can also

be distinguished by observers and the source of the noises invariably lies within the body of the patient. Some forms are also called *pulsatile tinnitus.*

2.   *Subjective tinnitus* generally describes a situation where the sounds heard by the patient are not audible to someone else, no matter what equipment may be used to try and detect them.

3.   Objective or subjective tinnitus can be further classified by how much it affects the patient. If the symptoms are so negligible (or happen so rarely) that the patient is often unaware of their occurrence, and it causes him or her but little bother, the condition is often described as *normal tinnitus.*

4.   On the other hand, *significant tinnitus* is used to describe a situation in which the disorder is either frequent and/or noticeable enough to interfere with the sufferer's daily routine.

Beyond objective or subjective, normal or significant, these general categories are not mutually exclusive.

1.   Objective *and* normal. In this case, the noises can be detected by others, but they

have hardly any effect on the patient.

2. Objective *and* significant. The noises can be independently confirmed and their effect upon the patient is great enough to cause discomfort, distress or worse.

3. Subjective *and* normal. The noises are only heard by the patient, but their effect remains minimal.

4. Subjective *and* significant. Only the patient can hear the noises and they have a considerable adverse effect on him or her.

Let us now look at the first two main types in greater detail.

Objective Tinnitus
(Somatosounds)

The human body is a very busy place with all kinds of processes taking place all the time: the heart beats, the lungs expand and contract, foodstuffs make their way along the intestinal track, joints move, blood courses through the veins and arteries, and so on. Many of these processes are far from silent and the sounds they make can often be readily detected by an independent observer using a stethoscope or other sound-amplification device at or near their source. The vast majority of people remain blissfully unaware of the noises made by their own body as it goes about its routine tasks for the following reasons:

⬦ The sources of many of the body's internal sounds lie in areas well insulated by surrounding muscles or other tissues which contain the vibrations created by the sounds and reduce their intensity outside the immediate area of their origin.

⬦ Despite the muffling effect of insulation that may be present, many inner-body sounds still have enough energy to fall within the audible range of human hearing by the time they reach the ears. However, because the brain has an amazing ability to ignore information that's not considered relevant, many (if not all) of these sounds will simply be "filtered" out.

Just as the brain can ignore "normal" bodily sounds, it also does an excellent job in recognizing when there is a sudden change. For example, someone with a slightly wheezy chest may be quite unaware of the sound this creates under normal circumstances. But if there is a change, the brain can stop its filtering of this particular sound, making it audible and thereby drawing the patient's attention to it. In some ways, making a previous inaudible sound perceivable can be compared to the protective aspect of pain, both serving to draw your attention to something that has gone wrong or that is no longer behaving normally.

Somatosounds generally result from one of three categories of disorders: vascular abnormalities, neurological disease or Eustachian tube dysfunction. They are usually described by the patient as a pulsing or clicking noise. Health practitioners can normally hear the sounds with the aid of listening devices such as stethoscopes, Toynbee tubes or Dopplers.

There are many possible sound sources within the body that can lead to objective tinnitus. Some of the main ones include:

⋄ *Circulation* has frequently been identified as a source of objective tinnitus. Especially likely to be heard is the flow of blood through the bigger vessels in the head or through the very small arteries that supply the ear, most specifically those leading to the inner ear. The heart is also a source of tinnitus noise and is comparatively easy to diagnose because the noise will almost invariably vary in close synchronization with the beat. Incidentally, it should be noted that being able to hear part of your circulatory system is by no means an indication that there is anything wrong. Despite that, it would be sensible to have your doctor do a general checkup.

⬧ Next to circulation, the *skeleton* is probably the most common source of sounds that result in objective tinnitus. Whereas all joints can potentially produce noise, the most likely offenders include bones in the jaw, neck, back and shoulders. Sometimes further investigation will discover that the "guilty" bones have suffered some deterioration from, for example, arthritis.

⬧ While *muscles* are a comparatively rare source of noises, those in the soft palate are an exception to this general rule, and tinnitus sounds have been clearly linked to their contraction.

Subjective Tinnitus

If no source can be identified for the noises heard by the patient, then the disorder will be described as subjective tinnitus. However, it's important to keep in mind that just because no inner body origin has been found to explain the noises, this is far from absolute proof that they don't exist. For example, some inner body sounds shown to be causes of objective tinnitus are extremely difficult to locate, even with the help of today's sophisticated amplifying instruments. Obscure sounds like these would probably never have been identified a few decades ago, and the patient would have been diagnosed as having subjective tinnitus. It's therefore not unreasonable to speculate that there are possibly other inner-body sounds so faint that their detection still remains beyond the power of modern gadgetry.

The phrase "subjective tinnitus" should never be interpreted as meaning the noises are *imagined* because almost certainly there is a physical cause for them, even if that cause is not producing sound but instead leads to what can only be called the *sensation* of sound. For example, the disorder can often be linked to damage in some area of the body. While the damaged area doesn't itself make a sound, it may nevertheless create nerve impulses that either the ear or the brain mistakenly recognizes as sound impulses. The origins of the subjective variety can often be traced to specific physical malfunction or damage.

Subjective tinnitus is more common than objective tinnitus and tends to affect older patients.

Significant or Not?

The dividing line between normal and significant tinnitus is often blurred because the extent to which someone is affected by the disorder depends more upon his or her reaction to the noises than upon how loud they are or appear to be.

Statistical surveys of tinnitus sufferers have often shown there can be quite a discrepancy between how loud or constant a sufferer says the noises are and how much he or she is affected by them. It would be totally wrong to assume that simply because a sufferer describes the noises he or she hears as "faint" or "occasional" they are therefore of little significance. On the contrary, some of the people most distressed by tinnitus report the sounds they hear as being quite faint. Conversely, other patients who report relatively loud tinnitus noises say they are not greatly bothered.

This lack of correlation between the loudness of tinnitus and how much it affects the patient occurs in both subjective and objective tinnitus. Incidentally, the fact that loudness doesn't necessarily bring proportionate distress has provided a very important clue as to how tinnitus (that cannot be cured) can still be alleviated considerably, as will be explained in later chapters.

Naturally, how frequently you hear the noise has a great bearing upon their impact. As might be expected, infrequent tinnitus is usually much easier to bear than if it is constant. Interestingly, some sufferers from intermittent tinnitus say it might bother them less if the noise was constant.

One patient explained: "It's bad enough when I hear the noises. But what's worse is not knowing *when* they may strike again. When I'm free of the noises for a good while, I begin to hope that I've been cured. Then the sounds come back, and that's such a letdown that I wish they had never gone away at all."

When and for how long tinnitus sounds are heard varies just as greatly as the nature of the sounds heard. At one extreme, some patients say their noises are with them constantly, with some even "hearing" them while they are asleep. Others say the sounds occur rarely, perhaps as infrequently as every few months. Most commonly, patients say the noises abate now and then with no obvious pattern to their presence or absence.

Finally, it should be noted that the level of tinnitus that a person endures can vary over time. Tinnitus that began as "normal" quite commonly worsens into "significant." More rarely, the reverse may also happen, and when it does it's usually because the sufferer has learned to adapt to his tinnitus rather than the condition itself having improved.

Incidentally, the phrase "normal tinnitus" is also used to describe a very temporary form of the disorder that just about everyone experiences now and then in a minor way. People who don't have tinnitus are still quite likely to hear "noises in their head" for a little while after having been exposed to very loud sounds like a rock concert. That kind of tinnitus, if that's what it really is, usually clears up of its own accord within minutes, or at worst, within an hour or so. However, there is evidence to indicate that repeated experiences of this kind are likely to predispose a person to the development of true tinnitus later.

The Noises of Tinnitus

While almost any kind of sound may be experienced by a tinnitus sufferer, the more common ones include:

- ◊ Ringing sounds, ranging from those resembling a telephone's shrill ring to more sonorous bell-like noises.

- ◊ Ill-defined sounds, somewhat like those made by a babbling brook.

- ◊ A hissing noise, usually quite high-pitched, resembling steam from the spout of a kettle coming to the boil.

- ◊ A buzzing noise, rather like that of swarming flying insects.

- ◊ Humming sounds in all their possible permutations, such as hums that sound like a muffled choir or like the background noise produced by a radio that's not tuned to a specific station.

⬥ Clicking sounds including those like the tapping of the keys of an old-fashioned typewriter or the sounds made by a car engine as it cools down after having been switched off. The clicks may follow a regular pattern or be totally random.

⬥ Whistling noises of all kinds ranging from human whistling to mechanical whistles, with both the pitch and the volume usually remaining fairly constant.

⬥ A throbbing noise, usually quite low in pitch.

⬥ Note for formatting: Cannot get diamond in right place

⬥ A noise that resembles a growl that never comes to a natural end but continues indefinitely.

⬥ Tweet-like sounds, almost like bird's chirping.

This list only covers a fraction of the noises that tinnitus sufferers have reported. In fact, it can be safely said that if you think of a sound—*any* sound—then it's almost certain that someone, somewhere experiences that sound as tinnitus. To further demonstrate just how varied tinnitus can be, here are some of the more unusual sounds as they were originally described by patients:

> "Sometimes I think what I'm hearing is the noise of the earth turning on its axis."

> "I keep hearing musical notes. All the notes have a very definite pitch and vary in length, just like those in a composition, but they never develop into anything remotely like a tune."

> "It's as though a group of very shrill-voiced children are shouting and yelling as they play their games in my head."

> "I can't describe the sound I hear, other than its very deep, very ominous and almost threatening."

> "It's just like being in the middle of what I imagine a railroad shunting yard to be like: the clatter of heavy steel wheels on rails; the hissing and puffing of steam engines; and the clanking of freight cars."

Although many people with tinnitus refer to noises that sound like those made by human voices, few report these noises as voices, generally choosing to describe them instead as being "voice-like." Yet some patients do say they hear quite distinct voices that, now and then, speak words that are recognizable and which may or may not make some sort of sense.

Some experts have speculated that more voices are heard by tinnitus sufferers than has been revealed by various research projects because patients may be reluctant to admit to "hearing voices" because this symptom is so strongly associated with certain forms of mental illness. However, judging by what has been reported by tinnitus sufferers who admit to hearing voices, the words are very different from those heard by mental patients. Tinnitus patients generally appear to hear random words, as though they were eavesdropping on a conversation. Whereas people with mental problems usually report that the voices are very clear, very definite, often speaking with great authority, as well as issuing commands and demands.

Stereo or Mono?

Depending on its causes, the sounds of tinnitus may be heard in both ears or only one. In fact, as we'll see later, this can be an important clue in determining what the underlying cause may be. Occasionally, the noises may shift from one ear to the other. Much more rarely, a patient may report that he or she "senses" the noises rather than "hears" them, the sensation appearing to be coming from somewhere within the head. Most commonly, tinnitus sufferers say they hear only one kind of noise, although some of its characteristics may change at different times—become louder or softer, shriller or deeper. Some patients, however, experience a whole gamut of different sounds, either separately or at times mixed together in total cacophony.

Summing Things Up

Tinnitus can manifest itself in an incredible variety of ways, with the possible permutations of its symptoms being virtually infinite. Although, according to the symptoms it produces, the disorder can be classified into several main categories, a patient's individual experience is almost certainly unique.

In the next chapter, we will be looking more closely at the various causes of tinnitus and how the risk of developing it can be reduced.

CHAPTER 4

Causes of Tinnitus & How to Prevent It

Note: In this chapter, we will use the word "cause" as it's generally understood by most people—something which brings about something else, the "something else" in this instance being tinnitus.

In some cases, it's possible to clearly establish a cause for tinnitus, like when it derives from taking certain medications or because the ear canal has become blocked by compacted ear wax. In most instances, however, the immediate cause is less obvious and may often be a matter of conjecture. A recent survey of nearly 1,000 tinnitus sufferers asked what they *believe* might have caused or triggered their tinnitus:

◊ Nearly a quarter of the respondents thought their tinnitus was due to previous exposure to loud noises.

◊ Just under a quarter attributed their problems to stress.

◊ One out of every five sufferers said their tinnitus was caused by having catarrh or being asthmatic.

Other causes frequently mentioned by patients include a history of hearing disorder (nearly 15 percent), accumulation of ear wax (six percent), and an operation not involving the ear (six percent). Other causes of lower incidence included migraines and headaches, as well as having suffered a heavy blow on the head.

When the same patients were asked to list events that occurred more or less at the same time as their tinnitus first became noticeable, the answers suggested other possible triggering factors:

◊ One in eight said the onset of the disorder followed a bad cold or influenza.

◊ Roughly ten percent said that loud noise had brought on the tinnitus; an equal number linked their condition to either

Meniere's disease or vertigo. Somewhat fewer patients said their tinnitus began when they became partially deaf.

◊   Other events mentioned frequently included an ear operation or ear infection (nearly nine percent), medical treatment with drugs or by injection for another problem (nearly nine percent), a blow to the ear or head (eight percent), preceding illness (nearly four percent). Interestingly, stress was mentioned by less than four percent.

Possible causes mentioned by relatively few sufferers included having their ears syringed to remove compacted wax (two percent), dental treatment that involved drilling (two percent), pregnancy (less than one percent), and menopause (less than one percent).

Just over 11 percent of respondents reported that their tinnitus started without any warning and they were unable to link its onset to any specific event.

These statistics, based on patients' personal viewpoints of their experiences, don't *prove* that these events actually caused the tinnitus. But they are certainly indicative. In most tinnitus cases, the origin is never determined. There may be very strong pointers suggesting what brought it on, but absolute proof of the root cause often remains elusive. However, there are many causes of tinnitus that can be clearly and unequivocally identified. We will now examine the main ones:

Noise

The National Institute of Deafness and Other Communication Disorders states that regular exposure to the following decibel levels (without protective gear) risks permanent hearing loss:

⋄ 110 decibels for more than one minute

⋄ 100 decibels for more than 15 minutes

⋄ 90 decibels for "prolonged exposure"

Examples of noises and their decibel levels include:

⋄ 140 decibels—rock concerts, firecrackers

⋄ 110 decibels—chain saw

⋄ 100 decibels—wood shop

⋄ 90 decibels—lawn mower, motorcycle.

Damaging noise can derive from unlikely places. A 2003 study of 11 children's toys by the Sight & Hearing Association found that nine of them produced more than 100 decibels. Chief offenders were a "talking" book called

Songs featuring the children's dinosaur character Barney and the Home Depot Workman's Screwdriver, which topped the noise chart at 115 and 112 decibels, respectively.

The damage that noise can cause to hearing can be divided into two major categories:

1. Damage that results from a single incident involving a very high level of noise. Typical examples of this are explosions or gunfire. Usually, but not always, the hearing impairment will manifest itself relatively soon, if not immediately. Extremely loud noises can totally destroy the organ of Corti in the inner ear, reducing it to fragments, and can sometimes trigger death.

2. Damage that follows repeated and prolonged exposure to noise, such as working in a noisy environment or spending many evenings in a noisy nightclub. This sort of damage usually takes a long time (years, even decades) before its effect becomes noticeable. Once again, the organ of Corti is usually affected with some of the hair cells destroyed, or the hairs themselves distorted, by the cumulative effect of noise exposure.

One of the difficulties with linking cause and effect in many types of hearing problems is that the disorder is often insidious, worsening so gradually that it may takes years before the patient becomes aware that something is wrong. Naturally, the way to prevent noise-induced hearing damage is to avoid loud noises. When this isn't possible, the following suggestions may help:

⋄ Wear the best possible ear protectors when operating noisy machines.

⋄ If your work environment is a noise one, make sure that all governmental regulations on noise levels are being met.

⋄ Consider wearing double ear protection. For example, use ear plugs *and* headsets when mowing the lawn and periodically turn the equipment off and check that the ear plugs are still properly seated.

⋄ Because sound damage is a function of both intensity and time, consider performing noisy activities in short spurts. For example, use the hedge trimmers for ten minutes, then take a five minute break and clean up what you've cut before trimming more.

⋄ When listening to music through earphones, always switch on the equipment and reduce the volume before placing the headset near your ears so that you won't be exposed to a sudden blast of high-intensity sound.

⋄ If rock concerts (or equally loud entertainment) are your pleasure, avoid being too
near the speakers.

⋄ If you are persistently and unavoidably exposed to loud noise, make sure you have your
hearing monitored at regular intervals. And
should you ever experience the slightest ringing in your ears, take this as a warning sign
and immediately seek professional advice.

The Aging Process

Even without the harmful effects of excessive noise,
it's a sad fact that hearing normally deteriorates
with the passing of years. Most commonly, high-
pitched sounds are no longer heard as clearly as
before, if at all. Initially, this loss doesn't matter all
that much for most people because the sounds they
can no longer hear are usually not important to
them. However, as the condition progresses and
begins to affect the middle range—that region between about 500 and 3,000 Hz, where most speech
falls—there may be difficulty in recognizing words
or parts of them.

In spoken English, most consonants are usually
pitched higher than vowels. Therefore, the first
noticeable sign of hearing loss may well be an
occasional inability to hear consonants. Another
classical indication of hearing loss is difficulty in

separating sounds, like trouble segregating one voice from others in general conversation involving several people.

It can be difficult to differentiate between "normal" hearing loss, due to the aging process, and that which has been exacerbated for other reasons. But as a general rule, the following can be expected (subject to great variations from individual to individual):

 ◊ The symptoms of normal hearing loss seldom become apparent before the age of sixty, although it will be the result of a very slow process that has been at work for decades. This hearing loss is invariably due to the degeneration of the hair cells and the nerve fibers in the organ of Corti, the damage being restricted to that area where the higher tones are perceived.

 ◊ Once the deterioration has become noticeable, it will appear to progress more rapidly. Relatively few people over seventy are still able to distinguish sounds much higher than the highest note on a piano.

Loudness Recruitment

A curious effect known as "loudness recruitment" normally accompanies hearing impairment that results from inner ear damage. Recruitment is characterized as:

⬥ Hearing will be poor when the sounds are of low intensity (intensity also being related to the distance separating the listener from the source).

⬥ Hearing will improve drastically as the intensity of the sounds increase (this improvement being much greater than that which would normally accompany the increase in intensity).

In other words, someone with loudness recruitment experiences larger variations in the volume of what he or she hears than those actually present in the sounds. Just why this phenomenon occurs is not yet fully understood. But some experts explain it as the brain increasing the ear's sensitivity across the currently audible range of frequencies, to make up for the loss of those frequencies which are no longer heard clearly. At first glance, recruitment may appear to be useful. But it actually creates more problems than it solves because it overemphasizes the normal volume variations in ordinary speech and can make it more difficult for an affected person to hear properly. Recruitment is one of the reasons why— if you slightly raise your voice when speaking to a hearing impaired person—you may be accused of shouting.

Recruitment is also believed to be a frequent contributor to tinnitus. The increased sensitivity it creates in some frequencies leads to the hearing of sounds whose intensity would otherwise have been too low to have been noticed. Although recruitment is difficult to explain, it can be compared to what happens when you turn up the volume control on a stereo: as the overall volume from the speakers increases, it also becomes easier to distinguish any background hiss or static that may be present.

Ear Wax

(*cerumen*)

Under normal circumstances, ear wax (produced by modified sweat glands in the skin lining our outer ear canals) fulfills several important purposes:

- ◊ It provides a barrier against possible infection, trapping dust and small foreign particles.

- ◊ It helps keep the ear canals supple while at the same time repelling excess moisture.

- ◊ It also acts as a "trap" for insects invading the outer ear, the intruders getting stuck on the wax before they can reach the ear drum and inflict damage.

Despite ear wax's beneficial role, it can be a source of hearing problems when it accumulates or becomes compacted or hardened. Generally, the ears will clear themselves of wax, but occasionally this automatic process fails to do a good enough job and the wax can then cause deafness and/or tinnitus. Fortunately, both conditions can be cured by the removal of the wax, something that can be accomplished in several ways. However, a warning: **Never introduce any instrument into your ears in an effort to clear wax.**

There are three good reasons for this admonition. Firstly, probing about in the ear is almost certainly going to compress what wax there may be there, making it less likely that nature will eventually clear it. Secondly, whatever object you use (be it a cotton swab or even a damp towel) is likely to irritate the ear canal's lining, making it secrete more wax than normal and so compound the problem. Finally, there's a good possibility that you may end up rupturing your ear drum!

Although there are various over-the-counter preparations you can buy to help shift recalcitrant wax, the best thing to do (if you have a hearing problem you believe is caused by wax) is to consult your doctor.

There are several methods for a health care professional to remove wax:

◇ The most commonly used devise is an ear syringe, a cylindrical metal instrument with a spout at one end and a plunger at the other. The syringe is filled with warm water, the spout applied to the ear and the plunger then pushed, propelling the water into the ear to wash away the wax

◇ A more modern version of the old-fashioned ear syringe is an instrument similar to the water picks used to massage gums or clear away food debris between teeth. Like the dental pick, this kind of syringe uses a jet of pulsating water. One big advantage of this method is the fact that the pick is small enough to allow observation inside the ear, allowing the operator to direct it exactly where needed.

◇ Perhaps the best way of removing wax is the "dry method" in which a delicate probe is used to pry it away and break it up, the fragments sucked up by a miniature vacuum pump. Unfortunately, this method is not available in all doctors' offices.

The following tips can help prevent wax from building up to the point where it becomes troublesome:

◇ Put a couple of drops of slightly warm— not hot!—olive oil in each ear about once a month to stop the wax from forming a solid plug. The easiest way to accomplish this is to stand in front of a mirror, tilt your head sideways, then use an eyedropper to drip the oil into your ear. Place a little cotton wool (make sure it's big enough not to be able to actually enter the ear canal, but is just jammed at its opening) in the outer rim of the ear for about twenty minutes to stop the oil from leaking out before the job is finished.

◊ Water entering the ear can swell any wax and compact it. To avoid this, wear earplugs when swimming; plug your ears with cotton wool before showering or shampooing; and make sure that your shower spray is never aimed directly at your ear opening.

While ear wax can be a direct cause of tinnitus, it has also been suggested that syringing compacted wax can set off the problem. Despite the vast amount of anecdotal evidence to support this idea, medical experts don't believe syringing leads to tinnitus, offering two possible explanations why the two may appear to be linked as cause and effect:

◊ The patient's hearing was already susceptible to tinnitus before the wax build-up and the disorder would have developed eventually in any case, its onset being purely coincidental.

◊ Wax (especially if it has collected on the ear drum rather than merely blocking the ear canal elsewhere) can create tinnitus. Once someone experiences the disorder, he or she becomes more aware of its symptoms and because of this increased awareness may now hear faint tinnitus that previously went unnoticed.

Otosclerosis

This is primarily a hereditary disorder that often develops from late adolescence then generally manifests itself in later life, when extra bone formation occurs in the inner ear. This overgrowth leads to restricted movement of the ossicles in the middle ear, the stapes usually being most severely affected, even to the point of becoming fixed to the oval window. Unless treated, the condition is progressive, leading to gradually deeper deafness as the transmission of sound vibrations becomes more and more impeded.

Tinnitus frequently accompanies developing otosclerosis, although it's also possible for a patient to have the two conditions simultaneously due to independent and separate causes. If tinnitus is present as a result of otosclerosis, then the noise it produces will usually be low-pitched.

Apart from tinnitus, another common symptom of otosclerosis hearing "distorted" sounds, with this distortion occurring long before loss of hearing becomes noticeable. The disorder is also frequently marked by patients claiming that their hearing is worst in quiet surroundings and appears more acute in noisy environments. Comparatively rarely, the condition may also be marked by vertigo.

Apart from using hearing aids to enhance the impaired sound recognition, otosclerosis can also be treated by *stapedectomy,* a surgical procedure that replaces the stapes with a small plastic piston that performs the same job. Stapedectomies are usually very successful in restoring hearing, but they don't always eliminate tinnitus.

Meniere's Disease

Usually affecting only one ear and relatively uncommon in people under the age of 50 years, Meniere's Disease (also known as *Meniere's Syndrome*) is a disorder of the inner ear with symptoms that include deafness, tinnitus, vertigo and vomiting.

The symptoms are brought on by a substantial increase in the amount of fluid in the semi-circular canals in the inner ear that helps control balance and determine body position. The extra fluid damages the canals and, at times, also the cochlea, thus interfering with sound perception and sometimes causing tinnitus. Unlike most other forms of deafness, the one that characterizes Meniere's Disease normally affect low frequency sounds, the loss usually being accompanied by loudness recruitment.

Most commonly, the first sign of the disorder is a sudden attack of vertigo, which is sometimes so severe that the patient may collapse. Attacks are occasionally preceded for a few days by discomfort or pain in the ear or tinnitus. How long attacks last and how often they occur varies greatly, but in most cases the deafness and tinnitus will persist between them.

The cause of Meniere's Disease remains unknown in about half of all cases, the others being attributed to a variety of factors including food allergies, congenital or acquired syphilis, low activity of the pituitary, adrenal or thyroid glands, diabetes, viral infection and high blood pressure. If a cause for the disorder can be identified, treatment will usually be addressed to rectifying the underlying problem. Other forms of treatment include drugs (notably *betahistine hydrochloride,* trade name *Serc*) which can lead to a reversal of the symptoms in the early stages of the disease. Left untreated, the condition invariably worsens, although the vertigo and the tinnitus may disappear as the deafness deepens or becomes total.

High Blood Pressure

There is a considerable amount of debate about the extent to which hypertension (higher than normal blood pressure) contributes to tinnitus. Certainly, if the hypertension leads to Meniere's Disease, then the link with tinnitus is proven. In many other instances, however, the connection is more tenuous, consisting mainly of the observation that many patients with tinnitus also have hypertension and that the former may improve when the latter is treated.

Whatever the general effects of hypertension on tinnitus, it can clearly influence tinnitus in two very specific ways:

1. Blood being pushed around the body at higher-than-normal pressure may create more intense sounds. If the tinnitus is of the pulsatile variety—the noises occur in synchronization with the pulse—then it seems likely that the louder the sounds made by the blood, the more likely these will be heard as tinnitus.

2. The tinnitus may be the result of the blood being pushed that much harder through the very fine arteries that supply the ear itself.

If you have tinnitus for no other obvious reason and are also hypertensive, then it may well be

51

that your hearing disorder will improve if you take steps to reduce your blood pressure. Equally, it seems logical—although not proven—that following a life-style that reduces the risk of hypertension may also reduces your chances of getting tinnitus.

Although it's beyond the scope of this book to delve deeply into hypertension, here are some suggestions that can help either prevent it or reduce the disorder if already present:

◊ Although severe hypertension may need drug treatment, milder instances can respond remarkably well to making simple life-style adjustments like keeping your weight down, getting more exercise, reducing your alcohol intake and stopping smoking.

◊ Mental stress and anxiety are strongly linked to raised blood pressure and these can also be factors influencing how much tinnitus affects you. Simple programs to reduce stress and promote relaxation are described in detail later in this book and these can provide a dual benefit by helping you cope better with tinnitus as well as reduce your blood pressure.

Apart from being a factor in tinnitus, hypertension also creates a substantially higher risk of eventually developing heart problems or having a stroke, and can also lead to many other serious diseases—all good reasons why it's a good idea to have your blood pressure checked regularly by your doctor.

High Levels of Adrenaline

Some experts believe that having high levels of adrenaline in your body can cause tinnitus. Adrenaline prepares your body for an emergency and it makes you much more reactive to the world around you—all senses are heightened, including hearing. If your body has too much adrenaline over too long a period, tinnitus can result.

Allergies

Some foods may trigger tinnitus. The chief offenders appear to include cheese, chocolate, red wine, soy, avocados, citrus and MSG. There is also controversy about whether the sugar substitute aspartame is linked to tinnitus, vertigo and other health problems. More details on this can be found in Chapter 6.

Tinnitus as a Symptom of Other Disorders

Tinnitus is also associated with a number of other diseases or conditions. Not uncommonly, tinnitus is the "presenting symptom"—the problem that compelled the patient to seek medical help in the first instance. While a complete list of disorders that include tinnitus as one of its symptoms would be virtually endless, here are some brief notes about the main ones:

Tumors—The word "tumor" merely indicates an abnormal swelling, usually due to an abnormal growth of tissue in or on part of the body and does not by any means indicate cancer (a tumor may be benign or malignant).

Acoustic neuroma is a kind of benign (noncancerous) tumor that creates tinnitus because it occurs in the fibrous sheet that covers the eighth cranial nerve, the one that links the inner ear with the brain. Tinnitus stemming from this cause is usually accompanied by vertigo because a branch of the affected nerve also carries the signals from the organs of balance in the ear. Almost invariably, only one ear is affected. While acoustic neuromas can be removed by surgery, this procedure does involve a risk of hearing loss and only produces noticeable relief from any associated tinnitus in about half the cases.

Glomous is another type of benign tumor that can cause tinnitus. It can be detected by a CAT scan and surgically removed. A warning: MRI, CAT and other scanning machines are invaluable with imaging, but are very loud and should only be used while wearing good protection.

Thyroid Problems—The thyroid gland controls the body's metabolic rate by releasing various hormones. Both an over-active or under-active thyroid—respectively *hyperthyroidism* or *hypothyroidism*—can be marked by tinnitus.

Diabetes—Already mentioned as a possible cause of Meniere's Disease, diabetes is a condition in which the body's cells fail to properly take in glucose as fuel due to a shortage of insulin. Various researchers have pointed out that a much higher proportion of tinnitus sufferers are also diabetics than might have been statistically expected.

Multiple Sclerosis (also known as *disseminated sclerosis*)—A chronic disease of the central nervous system, multiple sclerosis mainly affects young and middle-aged adults. MS, whose underlying cause remains unknown, causes damage in the myelin sheaths surrounding nerves in the brain and the spinal cord. If the disorder spreads to nerves linking the brain and the ears, then tinnitus may follow.

Meningitis—Tinnitus may be the first symptom of meningitis, an inflammation of the meninges (three connective tissue membranes that line the skull and vertebral canal) caused by viral or bacterial infection. Other common symptoms of meningitis include severe headache, rigidity of muscles, depleted appetite, and, in severe cases, convulsions. Treatment varies according to the cause, with bacterial meningitis responding to antibiotics and sulphonamides, while viral meningitis requires prolonged bed rest.

Head Injuries—As might be expected, injuries to the head (especially if surgery was required to deal with them) are often linked to immediate or later-onset tinnitus. Because of the number of variables involved, it's often unclear whether the tinnitus is a direct result of the injury or whether there already was a predisposition to the disorder.

Jaw Misalignment—Having misaligned jaw joints or jaw muscles can induce tinnitus as well as affect cranial muscles, nerves and shock absorbers in the jaw joint. There are dentists who specialize in what is called temporomandibular jaw misalignment.

Mercury Amalgam Tooth Fillings—British researchers June Rogers and Jacyntha Crawley say they have found a possible link between mercury tooth fillings and tinnitus.

Lyme Disease—This tick-borne disease, most common in the eastern United States, has been known to cause tinnitus as a side-effect.

Drugs—Medications with ototoxic side effects used to treat a variety of ailments can also produce tinnitus as a side-effect in susceptible people. For more information, see Chapter 6.

Summing Things Up

Tinnitus is caused by a wide-ranging variety of things and it can be difficult to identify which one is responsible in a given case. In the next chapter, we will discover how tinnitus is diagnosed and how treatment is matched to the cause.

CHAPTER 5

Diagnosis & Medical Treatments

Some purists argue that tinnitus is a symptom rather than a disorder or disease, and the noises associated with it are merely an indication that something is wrong. However, in general usage the word "tinnitus" covers a much wider area, denoting both symptom and disorder. The distinction can be an important one. Although one might say that someone is suffering from tinnitus, the fact may be that the patient has Meniere's Disease and tinnitus is merely one of its symptoms.

While on the subject of definitions, in this book we use the term "diagnosis" to describe the whole process involved in determining the nature of a disorder, taking into account many factors, including:

Symptoms—Problems the patient is aware of, such as being troubled by hearing noises which do not obviously match or are caused by sounds in the environment. The presence of one or more symptoms normally leads a patient to seek medical help.

Signs—Indications pointing to a particular disorder recognized by your doctor but which are not apparent to or recognized by the patient. For example, someone complaining of hearing noises may not be aware there is an accumulation of wax in the ear. But your physician will soon spot this as a sign of the underlying problem.

Medical background—Problems a patient may have had in the past can provide a vital clue to determining what's troubling him or her now, especially if the current difficulty appears to be repetition of a previous episode. To continue with the example, if a patient with compacted wax who complained of diminished hearing also disclosed that his ears had to be syringed in the past, it would be pretty obvious where the origin of the problem was likely to be found.

Results of laboratory or other tests—
Tests are determined by the initial examination findings, during which a tentative diagnosis may already have been reached and the tests merely a way for your doctor to confirm what he or she already suspects. In other instances, tests are required to exclude certain possible causes of symptoms, thereby reducing the number of conditions to consider. When tinnitus is the main or only symptom, tests of various kinds can play a major role in making a *differential diagnosis*—a diagnosis of a condition whose symptoms and/or signs also mark other conditions.

To start at the beginning of the medical process, someone experiencing tinnitus will almost invariably first turn to his or her family doctor. GPs will invariably tell you that it's very helpful if you take a list of all symptoms to your appointment, including details of your tinnitus bouts and what seems to have exacerbated the problem. You should also be prepared to share the complete list of medications you are taking and results from any hearing tests you've had in the past.

With tinnitus—as with so many other complaints—general practitioners have the unenviable task of acting as a clearinghouse, determining and judging whether a particular case lies within their own competence or if it needs to be treated by a specialist. Unless the problem is due to compacted ear wax or some other obvious and curable cause, the GP would usually refer a patient with ongoing and marked tinnitus to an Ear, Nose and Throat (ENT) specialist or otolaryngologist (oh-toe-lair-in-GAH-luh-jist).

It should also be noted that some GPs have to be coaxed somewhat before they will provide a referral, especially when the condition is mild. For those sufferers who might be reluctant to put pressure on their family doctor, it's well worth remembering that a hearing problem that remains less-than-fully diagnosed can only be expected to become worse. A curable condition can easily become an incurable one with the passage of time. It's therefore sensible to insist on being referred to a specialist if your tinnitus fails to improve after treatment provided by your GP.

Preparing for a Consultation

Having been referred to an ENT specialist, the chances are that you may well have to wait quite a while before your appointment. In the meantime, it's a good idea to keep up the notes that you made for your trip to the GP, jotting down details about new bouts of tinnitus, any new triggers you notice, etc.

It can also be useful to jot down other things which may or may not be connected with your tinnitus, such as what other health problems you are currently experiencing and whether there are any periods of high stress or bouts of anxiety and/or depression. Of particular importance, of course, is anything which occurs shortly before or at the same time that your tinnitus is at its worst. Equally important can be anything that seems to alleviate the severity of the problem.

To avoid the feeling of "I wished I'd thought of asking…" after your appointment, it's a good idea to write down some questions to ask the specialist, in case he or she doesn't cover them. At the end of the appointment, you can scan the questions to make sure you have all the answers you wanted. A few examples of these questions are:

1. Is treatment of tinnitus one of your specialties?

2. What treatments do you offer for tinnitus?

3. Are there any possible side effects from these treatments?

4. What is your success rate for tinnitus sufferers?

5. Are there any self-help methods you can suggest?

6. What is your experience with/views about alternative therapies and medicine for tinnitus treatment?

What Happens During a Consultation

Although individual consultants will have their own preferred approach, you can expect your initial examination to proceed more or less along set lines, beginning with an interview, then a physical examination and a brief check of some basic hearing functions. This will be followed perhaps by some more questions, after which you may be offered a diagnosis, possibly only a tentative one that will be subject to confirmation by further tests.

Questions You Are Likely to be Asked

After having taken down some general details, the consultant will then ask specific questions relating to your problems. Topics covered at this time will probably include:

⬦   Your general medical history, and possibly that of immediate family members as well.

⬦   What medications you are currently taking and which ones you've taken previously. This includes both prescribed medicines and those you've bought without a prescription.

⋄ If any jobs you've ever held might have created a special risk of hearing damage.

Then come questions dealing directly with the problem:

⋄ For how long have you been experiencing the difficulties?

⋄ Are both ears affected? And if so, to the same extent? If only one ear is affected, which one? Is the tinnitus "sensed" other places in your body other than in the ears? Is there or has there been discharge from the ears? If so, what form did it take?

⋄ Are the hearing difficulties accompanied by any pain or discomfort? If so, does this occur all the time or only occasionally? How severe?

⋄ Are the problems constant or only come up now and then?

⋄ Does the severity of the condition vary greatly over time?

⋄ Did the problem come on all at once? Or was there a period over which it developed gradually, perhaps even almost imperceptibly?

What does it sound like? Is it high-pitched, low-pitched or just a vague noise without any apparent specific pitch?

⋄   Have you ever experienced vertigo (dizziness)? If so, do you suffer constantly, frequently or only occasionally? How severe is the dizziness? Does it merely make you feel somewhat unstable or does it lead to actual loss of balance?

Depending upon his or her tentative conclusions, the consultant may ask further questions. These might include:

⋄   Have you yourself noted any events which seem to make the problem worse or better?

⋄   To what extent does the problem affect you other than just physically? Does it make you anxious or depressed? If so, how severe is the anxiety or depression?

⋄   Do you frequently have severe headaches or migraines? Any problems with your eyesight, such as double vision, blurring, loss of peripheral vision? Any difficulties in controlling your limbs? Any numbness or reduced sensation in any part of your body? Any difficulties with your speech? Do you have lapses of memory?

In most cases, the consultant will have a pretty good idea about the likely cause of the problem once these questions are answered. But almost invariably, no opinion will be offered at this time. He or she will proceed directly to the next stage.

Physical Examination

Depending upon the circumstances, this may be divided into three areas: an examination of aspects of your body that aren't obviously thought of as being linked to hearing difficulties; an examination of the ears; and some simple tests to determine how well your hearing works.

While tinnitus may be the specific reason why you've been referred to a consultant, the examination will nevertheless cover all aspects of your hearing. The reason for this is simple: tinnitus is frequently accompanied by deteriorating hearing, but this impairment is often so slight (or its onset so gradual) that the patient hasn't noticed. But the existence or non-existence of partial deafness will provide strong evidence as to the likely cause of the tinnitus, many forms of which can improve dramatically once any underlying deafness has been treated.

If the consultant thinks that your hearing problem may be a symptom of some other disease, he or she will look for signs that might confirm the presence of another disorder. For example, should the doctor think your tinnitus stems from hypertension, he or she will check your blood pressure.

In the absence of the likelihood of another underlying problem, the consultant will proceed directly to a visual examination of the ear, this naturally being limited to the outer ear. Once again, how he or she does this may vary, but generally this is what will happen:

⬥ The consultant will usually begin by looking carefully at each auricle, the part of the outer ear that lies outside the head, pressing and probing gently for signs of inflammation, discharge or undue tenderness.

⬥ He or she will then inspect your ear canals, almost certainly using an *auriscope* (also known as an *otoscope*), a hand-held device that includes a funnel (speculum) that is introduced into the ear, a source of light and an array of lenses that provide a clear view of the inside of the outer ear. Alternatively, the visual inspection may be carried out with the aid of a microscope. Either way, the consultant will be looking for evidence of excessive wax and inflammation or discharge, as well as anything indicating damage to the ear drum or ear canal.

⬥ Finally, the consultant will check whether your Eustachian tubes are opening and closing properly. You will be asked to you to blow your nose while keeping your nostrils shut, an action that should cause the Eustachian tube (leading from the pharynx to the middle ear) to admit air from the outside. Then you'll be asked to swallow, an action that allows for the escape of air from the middle ear.

Once the visual examination is completed, the next thing will almost certainly be a series of simple hearing tests. Just what these may consist of can vary greatly. Some consultants choose to carry out a whole battery of tests themselves, while others let technicians carry out whatever tests may be required.

From these tests, your consultant will be able to determine whether your problem falls into the *conductive* or *sensorineural* category. Conductive hearing loss occurs when sound waves are prevented from passing to the inner ear and is caused by a variety of problems including earwax buildup (cerumen), punctured eardrum or ear infection (otitis media). This type of hearing loss can often be corrected by medical or surgical treatment). Sensorineural hearing loss is caused by damage to the auditory nerve or hair cells in the inner ear and is generally caused by aging, noise, illness, injury, toxic medications or an inherited condition. Hearing aids are particularly useful for people suffering from sensorineural hearing loss.

After the Exam

Once the examination is completed, your consultant is quite likely to have a few more questions. Usually, these will be aimed mainly at confirming the findings; occasionally, he or she may ask you to explain in greater detail some of the things you touched upon briefly during the first stage of the consultation. In most cases, you will then be offered a diagnosis, although that may be reserved until further tests have been completed.

Audiometry

Although any form of checking someone's hearing could be called *audiometry,* the term is normally used to describe tests involving electrical apparatus.

Modern-day audiometers test hearing in great and comprehensive detail. As you'll recall from a previous chapter, the range of frequencies used by human speech is a comparatively narrow band of those that someone with perfect hearing can perceive. Although it may be desirable to be able to hear as wide a range of frequencies as possible, the fact is that hearing is generally considered adequate for most purposes providing it is sufficiently sensitive to those frequencies covered by speech.

There's another very practical reason why this band of frequencies is the one most taken into account: most hearing aids are designed in such a way that they will only bring substantial improvement within that range. What this means is that while any loss of hearing in other frequencies may be indicative of the nature of the problem, the testing of hearing will generally concentrate on those frequencies lying between 250 and 8,000 Hz, with an even narrower range than that only being checked sometimes.

Hearing is tested with an *audiometer*, an instrument capable of synthesizing different tones at varying frequencies at various levels of intensity. The sound—usually a pure tone somewhat like a continuous tuneless whistle— is delivered to the patient through close-fitting earphones that exclude ambient noise, or possibly through loudspeakers.

Two different but inter-connected aspects of hearing are measured during testing—what frequencies can be heard and how loud the sound has to be (at different frequencies) before it becomes audible. The results are plotted on two graphs (one for each ear) called *audiograms*. At the left side of each audiogram is a descending scale—usually ranging from 130 to 10 dB—where hearing sensitivity is recorded. At the bottom of the graph is another scale, this one covering the frequency range from just below 125 to just over 8,000 Hz.

During testing, the technician uses the audiometer to send out tones of varying frequencies and volumes. The patient signals—usually by pressing a bell button, but possibly verbally—when he or she detects the incoming sound. Most commonly, the test will begin with tones in the upper middle range—say between 500 and 4,000 Hz. Typically what happens is the following:

⬥ In order to test sensitivity, a signal at a given frequency (say 500 Hz) is transmitted to the patient at various levels of loudness so the lowest level where the sound is heard can be identified. Depending upon the technician, this may be done in two different ways: by gradually reducing the intensity until the sound is no longer heard; or by starting with a volume setting that is so low that the sound will almost certainly be inaudible and then gradually raising the volume until it's heard. Alternatively, a combination of both methods may be used to pinpoint exactly what the patient's threshold of audibility is for a particular pitch.

⬥ The same testing will repeated for the other frequencies, and the whole series will then be repeated for the other ear.

What emerges from this test is a clear graphic indication of the hearing in each ear, represented on its respective audiogram as a line. Peaks show where the hearing in a given frequency is good; troughs indicate where hearing is deficient.

Audiograms, of course, need expert interpretation. But as a generality, good or acceptable hearing—broadly defined as hearing that will probably not be improved to any great extent by a hearing aid—will be indicated by the following:

◊ Sounds in the frequencies ranging from 125 to 3,000 Hz should be heard when their loudness is 20 dB or less. Most commonly, however, these will be perceived at 10 dB or even less.

◊ While sounds above 3,000 Hz generally need to be louder than the above before they are heard, there usually is a fairly steep drop-off in sensitivity in the higher pitches. The extent to which the drop-off in the higher frequencies is considered as "normal" is partly based upon the subject's age.

Some of other factors that will be taken into account when interpreting the audiograms:

◊ The age of the subject. Some loss of hearing—not necessarily limited only to high frequencies—is part and parcel to the natural aging process in all of us.

◊ If some of the readings for the high-middle frequencies fall into the 20 dB plus range, then how many of them do so? For example, merely discovering that *one* ear provides less than fully adequate hearing at only *one* frequency is usually not all that significant and doesn't, in and of itself, suggest that the patient will benefit from a hearing aid. If the same defect is markedly noted in a group of adjoining frequencies, then a hearing aid is more likely to help.

Incidentally, it needs to be pointed that audiograms use "0" to indicate the threshold of hearing. This threshold is based upon a standard obtained by studying the hearing of a large number of young people with totally healthy hearing. Despite that, the threshold mark remains an arbitrary one. Many people whose hearing is perfectly fine for everyday purposes fail to hear *any* frequencies at such a low level, requiring the sound to often be at least five, ten or even more decibels louder. There are some people whose hearing is so very sensitive that they can detect some frequencies at lower intensities than 0 dB. A standard audiogram starts at -10 dB so that these quite rare occurrences can be recorded without the line going off the chart.

Additional Tests

In most cases, a standard audiometer test will be enough to provide all the necessary data to enable a diagnosis. But occasionally, a *bone conduc-*

tion test is also requested. This is similar to the test described above, except that the sounds generated by the audiometer are not transmitted to the subject's ears through earphones but are instead sent to the mastoid bone through a small device clamped against it.

Within this device, sound vibrations created by a miniature loudspeaker connected to the audiometer are translated into mechanical vibrations, applied directly against the bone via a tiny piston. Bone is an excellent transmitter of vibrations and those produced by the piston are received by the cochlea (both of them, in fact, although the one nearest to the piston will perceive the vibrations much more clearly than the other).

As this system of transmitting sound vibrations bypasses both the outer and middle ear, tests carried out this way will pinpoint exactly what sounds can be heard by the cochleas and/or transmitted via the hearing nerves. Much valuable information about the source of the problem can be gained by comparing audiograms obtained in the usual manner with those resulting from bone conduction testing.

Additionally, many other kinds of tests can be carried out should the circumstances warrant. The main ones include investigations to determine: how easily and smoothly the ear drum and the ossicles respond to vibrations; the air pressure in the middle ears (this providing information about whether the Eustachian tubes are working properly); and how well the stapedial reflex is working (the automatic reflex that helps protect hearing against very loud sounds in excess of 80 dB). The latter test is carried out by tensing a small muscle linked to the third ossicle and thus reducing the intensity of the sound conducted further along the lie to the cochlea.

The Diagnosis

When all tests have been completed, your consultant will be in a position to make his diagnosis. At that time, there will be two main possibilities:

1. The tinnitus appears to be due to (or is a symptom of) some other underlying problem which can be cured or helped by medical treatment, such as inflammation, otosclerosis, thyroid problems or Meniere's Disease. In this case, the relevant medical treatment will be offered with the hope that, as well as clearing up the underlying disorder, it will also cure or reduce the tinnitus. A medically treatable condition will, however, only be found in about five percent of the cases.

2. As happens in about 95 per cent of instances of tinnitus, the examination and tests will fail to reveal any medically treat-

able cause for the disorder, other than the fact that the disorder is also accompanied by hearing that is somewhat failing.

Depending upon your point of view, the fact that medical investigation usually fails to find a medically treatable cause in about 19 out of 20 cases of tinnitus can be seen as either good or bad news. To look at the bright side, this means that most instances of tinnitus are not the result of another disease whose eventual consequences may be even more dire. The bad news, of course, is that most cases of tinnitus are not going to be cured by medical treatment. This, however, must not be interpreted as meaning that medically untreatable tinnitus cannot be treated or even possibly "cured" to the extent that its effects are no longer noticeable. It simply means that the help for the condition will not come in a form that can be provided by medication or surgery.

The American Tinnitus Association offers a referral service for medical doctors, audiologists and other tinnitus specialists. To locate service in your area, call the ATA's toll-free number: (800) 634-8978.

Drug Treatments for Tinnitus

Just what non-medical help is available to ease tinnitus will be covered in depth in the next few chapters. However, before going on, we will take a brief look at some medical treatments (excluding those for specific conditions covered in the previous chapter) that have achieved varying degrees of success in making tinnitus more bearable. Seldom are drugs prescribed just for tinnitus alone; many of those mentioned have been mainly used in trials and the results not always fully confirmed by further studies.

⋄   *Barbiturates* (such as Amytal) are mainly used as sedatives, to counteract insomnia, and to reduce anxiety, but have also proven of value in relieving tinnitus. Despite various studies, it remains less than clear how they soothe tinnitus—it could be due to a reduction in stress and anxiety or a lessened perception of tinnitus, or perhaps a combination of both these factors. Whatever may be the true explanation, barbiturates do work for some tinnitus sufferers.

   However, doctors are often reluctant to prescribe these drugs. Firstly, patients can quickly become dependent on them. Secondly, the beneficial effects may soon decrease as tolerance sets in. The combination of these two factors all too often leads to situations where the drug does little to aid the problem for which it was prescribed but is still prescribed to postpone the problems that may accompany withdrawal. Additionally, the long-term use of barbiturates can lead to severe side effects, including permanent liver damage.

◊ Several studies have been done on the effect of *lignocaine* (also known as lidocaine) upon tinnitus. Normally these drugs are used as local anesthetics or for regularizing erratic heart rhythms. But it was found that injections of lignocaine and related drugs can bring substantial relief from tinnitus, even clearing it up completely in some patients. Unfortunately, the drug has to be administered intravenously and the relief is short-lived, most commonly lasting only a few hours. What's more, the drugs can lead to serious side effects, including confusion and convulsions. Due to this, most experts have concluded that these drugs are not a practical treatment method for tinnitus. Further research continues, much of it concentrating on a form of lignocaine that can be taken orally.

◊ *Tranquillizers* (such as diazepam or lorazepam) are quite frequently prescribed for tinnitus sufferers. It's not believed these drugs have any affect whatever on the disorder itself, their value being confined to enabling the patient to cope better with the symptoms.

Although exact figures are lacking, it's thought that a sizeable number of tinnitus sufferers are receiving regular prescriptions for tranquillizers.

Various studies have reported greatly conflicting evidence about the value of such treatment. For example, one research project found that two-thirds of tinnitus sufferers were helped by taking a minor tranquillizer. Other studies have concluded that the benefits of such a regime are outweighed by the risks of side effects and possible dependence. It seems the extent to which tranquillizers can help is an individual matter. Currently available research results strongly suggest these drugs are most likely to be of substantial benefit when a) the tinnitus is quite severe; and b) the patient has other problems related to stress and/or anxiety.

◊ *Tricyclic* and related antidepressants often exacerbate tinnitus, but paradoxically may help some sufferers. Once again, it's less than clear just how these drugs soothe tinnitus. Some experts believe that this may be due to an anticonvulsive effect. Others, considering the links between stress, anxiety and depression, find a simpler explanation. One intriguing aspect of these antidepressants is that they can help reduce oral and facial pain, leading some researchers to speculate about how they may affect the nerves involved in the hearing process.

◊ *Anti-convulsants* like carbamazepine (Tegretol), phenytoin (Dilantin), primidone (Mysoline) and valproic acid (Depakene) have shown some effectiveness in reducing tinnitus. Some of these drugs can have serious side effects that require careful monitoring via blood chemistry and other tests.

◊ One medication which deserves special mention because of its apparent effectiveness and safety in relieving tinnitus symptoms is *alprazolam* (brand name Xanax), a medication normally used for treating anxiety associated with depression. It's also widely used to treat panic disorders. A double-blind study of 20 patients in the Portland, Oregon area suffering from tinnitus showed 76 percent of the participants experienced at least a 40% reduction in tinnitus symptoms after using this drug. The study was conducted by Robert M. Johnson, Ph.D.; Robert Brummett, Ph.D.; Alexander Schleuning, M.D. (Arch Otolaryngol Head Neck Surg. 1993: 119:842-845).

However, the doctors did make some provisos at the conclusion of the study. They said that while alprazolam appears to be beneficial in treating some patients with tinnitus, long-term use of a benzodiazepine is not recommended. Patients are usually prescribed this medication for a maximum of four months, after which the dose needs to be reduced and then discontinued for at least a month. The doctors also pointed out that, for some patients, continuing at a very low dosage was sufficient to keep the tinnitus at a low level. In addition, the doctors warned that it's important to regulate the prescribed dosage of alprazolam since individuals differ considerably with regard to sensitivity to this medication. You'll have to visit your doctor to get a prescription for this medication.

Another treatment that you should ask your doctor about is *Dimethyl sulfoxide* (DMSO), a colorless hygroscopic liquid obtained from lignin, used as a penetrant to convey medications into tissue. In a study published in the *Annals of the New York Academy of Sciences*, a DMSO solution containing anti-inflammatory and vasodilatory compounds was applied every four days to the external auditory canals of the ears of 15 tinnitus sufferers. At the same time, they were also given an intramuscular injection of DMSO. After a month, nine patients said their tinnitus had disappeared—and it didn't return during the one-year observation period. Of the remaining six patients, two said their tinnitus was lessened and four said that it became only an occasional problem instead of permanent (cold temperatures seemed to be the main factor causing it to return).

Other Medical Treatments

◇ *Cochlear Implants*—Designed for people with little or no hearing, these surgically implanted devises do offer tinnitus relief for some patients. However, this is a risky choice, as some patients have reported that this therapy actually worsens their tinnitus.

◇ *Dental Treatment*—Damage to the Temporomandibular joint (TMJ), which can result in jaw clicking, ear pain and tinnitus, can often be effectively treated by a dentist.

◇ *Electrical Stimulation*—This experimental treatment involves transmitting electrical energy to the cochlea via electrodes placed near the ear. While some success has been reported with this treatment, there have also been reports of the tinnitus getting worse.

Summing Things Up

We have covered in this chapter just a few of the treatments that have been tried for tinnitus. Unfortunately, none has, to date, proven itself sufficiently effective to be described as a treatment of choice. This doesn't mean that drugs and other therapy may not provide valuable relief for many tinnitus sufferers, just that the results are often unpredictable and that any benefits have to be carefully weighed against the risks of side effects and dependence that any long-term drug regime usually involves.

In the next chapter, we will look at other ways of reducing the impact of tinnitus, especially by avoiding or reducing our exposure to things that may either trigger it or make it worse.

CHAPTER 6

Reducing the Impact of Tinnitus

While medical treatments are, unfortunately, of only limited help to a minority of tinnitus sufferers, there are many other ways in which the impact of the symptoms can be substantially reduced, even possibly eliminated. These non-medical forms of help fall into three main categories:

1. The identification (and subsequent avoidance) of those things that may set off symptoms and/or make them worse.

2. Electronic devices, such as hearing aids and tinnitus maskers, that reduce the ef-

fect of tinnitus either by improving the hearing as a whole or minimizing tinnitus by introducing other sounds that have a tendency to "cancel" it out. For more details, see the next chapter.

3. Different ways of altering how strongly the sufferer reacts to tinnitus, hopefully leading to a lessened perception of the noises and thereby making the disorder more acceptable and less intrusive or disabling. These approaches, which usually rely heavily on stress and anxiety reduction, are closely interwoven with preventing the symptoms from arising in the first place. (See chapters 8 and 9.)

In this chapter, we will concentrate on those things that for many people make tinnitus worse, if not necessarily causing it. However, before we proceed, a note of explanation and caution is in order:

Subjective tinnitus invariably manifests itself in a very individual way with probably no two sufferers experiencing it absolutely identically. Equally individualistic are the things that can make the disorder better or worse for a given sufferer. This means that the suggestions and recommendations that follow will not work in every case. For example, while giving up smoking will probably help most sufferers, there are those for whom the stress of nicotine withdrawal may perhaps precipitate worse symptoms than ever before. Readers are therefore strongly urged to consider the following facts in the light of their own individual circumstances.

Food Allergy and Tinnitus

There is little doubt that many instances of tinnitus are worsened by eating certain foods, either a side effect from an allergic reaction to the food or a substance in the food causing a direct effect. There are some foods that have repeatedly been identified by tinnitus sufferers as worsening their symptoms and it would certainly be worth trying to avoid these dishes for some time to see whether or not that makes any appreciable difference in your case. Incidentally, we also mention foods that are linked to hearing loss in general, as tinnitus and hearing loss often occur together and improving hearing often reduces accompanying tinnitus. Foods most likely to be "offenders" include:

⬦ Coffee, tea and other drinks (such as colas) that contain caffeine, a powerful stimulant. Although caffeine's initial effect is that of a pick-me-up, this temporary boost is soon followed by a letdown. Researchers have found that this see-sawing between highs and lows can heighten anxiety and bring on depression in susceptible people. Decaffeinated coffee and tea appear to have no effect on tinnitus.

87

◇ A similar effect to that of caffeine has been attributed to cocoa, which is mainly found in chocolate, pastries, cakes and chocolate drinks. It's also often one of the ingredients of processed and/or packaged foods.

◇ Foods high in saturated fats have also been implicated. These, of course, are likely to raise your cholesterol level, possibly leading to hypertension, a condition strongly associated with tinnitus. Additionally, several studies have confirmed a link between sensorineural hearing loss and high levels of blood fats. This is probably due to high blood-fat levels causing hearing loss by restricting the supply of oxygen and nutrients to the inner ear. Further research has shown that following a diet that's low in saturated fats provides some protection against hearing loss and can even help bring about improvement for those who have already lost some hearing.

◇ Alcohol. The evidence about the adverse effect of alcohol in tinnitus is rather mixed. Generally, studies have found that for most sufferers, drinking alcoholic beverages tends to make the condition worse. But some patients report that alcohol improves matters for them, albeit only temporarily. It's worth noting that alcohol, seen by many people as a stimulant, is in fact a sedative and that could explain why it may be beneficial in small amounts for patients whose tinnitus is strongly linked to anxiety or stress.

◊ Cutting down your salt intake may reduce tinnitus, according to many sufferers. Remember that many processed foods also have a high salt content and seek to avoid these.

◊ A high intake of sugar, say researchers, can be instrumental in bringing about hearing loss. Scientists believe that this happens because sugar stimulates the release of adrenaline, and this can reduce the oxygenated blood supply to the inner ear by constricting the small arteries that supply it. Improvements in hearing, as well as occasionally reduced tinnitus, have been reported by some people after reducing their intake of sugar and other refined carbohydrates.

◊ Food allergies in general have been strongly linked to frequent bouts of middle-ear inflammation, a disorder which, if left untreated, can eventually cause damage to the ossicles. In a major study involving more than a hundred subjects with frequent or chronic ear infections, it was found that more than three-quarters of them were allergic to one or more common foods. When the implicated foods were withdrawn from their diets, three out of four of the subjects had either no further ear infections or only experienced them very occasionally. The most common foods creating an allergic reaction were wheat and soybean products, milk, eggs and peanuts.

The specific foods mentioned above are those which have often been implicated in tinnitus. However, judging from patient accounts, just about any food could be a source of trouble. If you suspect food allergies are making your symptoms worse, begin by eliminating a few of the ones listed above for a week or two. If that makes no difference, then eliminate another lot for a while, continuing in this manner until at one time or another you've temporarily eliminated all of them. Should none of this help, try keeping a diary of the foods you eat and the severity of your tinnitus. Do this for a couple of weeks and then look back on your entries, analyzing and comparing them. If you're lucky, you may spot a direct correlation between a particular food and worsening symptoms.

However, the food-tinnitus link is often not as obvious as this and you need bear in mind that there could be a substantial period of time separating a food "cause" and its resultant effect. As this time-lag can be three days or even longer, it may require a lot of patient detective work before a pattern reveals itself.

Foods that May Help

Several nutritional deficiencies have been associated with some kinds of sensorineural hearing loss and, by extension, with the development of tinnitus. While there is no scientific proof that ensuring that your diet contains these nutrients will alleviate either hearing loss and/or tinnitus, this is obviously a sensible thing to do. If you decide to make up a shortfall of any nutrient by taking supplements, you should first consult your doctor.

Associated with hearing loss are deficiencies of:

⬥ **Vitamin A (Retinol)**—Good natural sources of this vitamin include fresh vegetables (especially green or yellow), cod liver oil, liver, milk and butter.

⬥ **Vitamin D (Cholecalciferol)**—Good natural sources of this vitamin include cod liver oil, egg yolk, margarine and cream. Vitamin D is also produced by synthesis within the skin when exposed to sunlight.

⬥ **Iron**—Good natural sources of iron include meat, oysters, liver, chicken and turkey. Note, however, that too much iron can be just as harmful as too little because an over-abundance of the mineral can increase the risk of arterial disease and heart attacks.

◊ **Zinc**—Good natural sources of zinc include lamb, pork, oysters, herrings, pumpkin seeds, eggs, milk, beans, yeast and brewer's yeast.

Drugs that Could Worsen Matters

Both prescribed drugs as well as those contained in preparations available without a prescription can contribute to creating deafness and/or tinnitus, whether temporarily or permanently. Additionally, many drugs that by themselves would do no harm can interact with other drugs (taken at the same time for other conditions) to create a new set of potential side effects. This possibility is one more good reason why you should always keep your doctor fully informed about any non-prescribed medication you're taking.

During one recent international symposium on tinnitus, experts listed more than a hundred drugs whose use has been implicated in either creating or worsening tinnitus, with about half of them also linked to hearing loss. It needs to be emphasized, however, that most of these drugs only affected the hearing of a very small minority of patients who took them, and that problems with many of these medications only arose when they were taken in much higher dosages than normal. What's more, a person's reaction to a given drug is often highly individualistic, just as a food allergy can be.

Commonly used drugs that have been identified as causing and/or contributing to tinnitus include:

- ◊ **Aspirin.** This most common of all pain-killers is notorious for its ability to create tinnitus, usually of the high-pitched variety. But for this to happen, the dosage usually has to be quite high% perhaps several times that recommended for ordinary usage—and the medication taken for some time. While it is not believed that the occasional use of aspirin at a moderate dosage will heighten the risk of tinnitus, it's obviously sensible to avoid this particular analgesic if you have hearing problems. Having said that, it also needs to be pointed out that some patients with well-established and quite severe tinnitus have reported that taking aspirin has *helped* reduce their symptoms.

- ◊ **Ibuprofen and indomethacin.** There is some evidence, sparse but accumulating, that these drugs, commonly used to control mild to moderate pain and inflammation in rheumatic disease and other musculoskeletal disorders, may lead to tinnitus or worsen the affliction when already present.

⋄ **Antibiotics.** These are medicines that destroy or inhibit the growth of micro-organisms and are commonly used to treat a wide range of conditions arising from bacterial of fungal infection. Although these drugs have literally proven to be lifesavers on countless occasions, they too have been implicated in tinnitus, although there is no accepted scientific explanation as to why this happens. Nevertheless, the accumulated anecdotal evidence from tinnitus sufferers is so great that there is little doubt that antibiotics can trigger tinnitus or make it worse.

⋄ **Antidepressants.** The role of antidepressants in tinnitus is a curious one. As has already been indicated, they can be a vital part of the treatment when the tinnitus is caused (or worsened) by anxiety, stress and depression. In fact, there are now many experts who believe that antidepressants are a better overall therapy for some forms of anxiety, including those specifically linked to tinnitus, than tranquillizers. On the other hand, there is plenty of evidence to show that antidepressants can create tinnitus, the condition usually (but not always) disappearing when the drugs are discontinued. The only way to find out whether antidepressants will help is by trying them (at the suggestion of your doctor). Naturally, tell your doctor immediately if your symptoms worsen. By the way, should you be on a prescribed course of antidepressants, do not discontinue these without your doctor's prior approval, as serious side effects can occur during uncontrolled withdrawal.

⬥ **Diuretics.** Also linked to producing or exacerbating tinnitus are diuretics, drugs that increase the volume of urine produced by promoting the excretion of salts and water from the kidneys. The more potent diuretics are used to reduce salt and water retention in disorders of the heart, kidney, lungs and liver; milder preparations are used to treat high blood pressure as well as reduce intraocular pressure in glaucoma.

⬥ **Quinine.** Only rarely used nowadays, quinine was once commonly prescribed to treat and prevent malaria, an infectious disease caused by the presence of parasitic protozoa in the red blood cells. One of the drug's well-established side effects is *cinchonism*, a poisoning caused by too high a dosage of quinine (or similar alkaloids) and whose symptoms include ringing noises in the ears, as well as dizziness and poor balance.

◊ **Cannabis.** Although not a medicine in this country, the drug cannabis (also known as marijuana) may worsen preexisting cases of tinnitus. Because its use is illegal in the United States and therefore largely unrecorded, the evidence linking cannabis to tinnitus is mainly circumstantial. However, there is no doubt that tinnitus-like experiences can be part of marijuana's euphoric effects. There is less certainty about whether such tinnitus may eventually become permanent.

Smoking

Experts agree that smoking is likely to worsen existing tinnitus, but there is greater skepticism about whether the habit makes any sizeable contribution to increasing the risk of developing the condition.

Several studies have shown that smokers with moderate to severe subjective tinnitus have often reported an improvement in their symptoms after they stopped smoking for some time. There is, however, another side to the coin—some smokers found that stress caused by trying to give up smoking made their tinnitus worse. It's open to speculation whether their symptoms might have improved had they persevered long enough with their attempt to reach the point where the long-term benefits began to outweigh temporary side effects.

If you do quit smoking, there is a very good chance that this will improve your tinnitus, as well as the additional bonus of greatly reducing your risk of developing many serious diseases. Incidentally, it needs to be added that non-smoking tinnitus sufferers have often reported that their condition is worsened when they are exposed to other people's smoke.

Reducing the Harmful Impact of Loud Noises

Various ways to protect your hearing by avoiding loud noises were mentioned in Chapter 4, but these recommendations dealt mainly with noises that were under your own control. Unfortunately, in today's overcrowded towns and cities, many of us are subjected to noises stemming from seemingly uncontrollable sources. As existing tinnitus is often aggravated by certain noises in the environment, here is a brief summary of what steps you can take to reduce noises that you consider to be a nuisance. Please bear in mind that a *reasonable* level of surrounding noise is part and parcel to modern living.

1. If your neighbors are the source of the noise—things like loud music and barking dogs—then the first thing you should do is approach them politely, explain the problem and hope that things quiet down. Should this approach fail to bring results, your next step is contacting the local police to discuss your options.

2. An alternative approach, although fraught with possible legal pitfalls, is to take civil action against the noise maker. Civil actions can become very expensive and you should certainly seek legal advice before embarking on this course.

Summing Things Up

Most of the information in this chapter was aimed at showing how you can reduce the severity of your tinnitus symptoms by following some simple recommendations. For many sufferers, the relief obtained from these self-help suggestions may be enough to make their condition considerably more acceptable. However, there are other ways of reducing the impact of tinnitus, including "masking" its noises with other sounds, as we'll discover in the next chapter.

CHAPTER 7

Hearing Aids & Tinnitus Maskers

As deficient hearing and tinnitus often go hand-in–hand, one logical step towards possibly alleviating tinnitus is to improve the hearing by using an electronic aid. While not all people with tinnitus also have hearing loss that can be helped by a hearing aid, many of them do. In those cases, artificially restoring hearing through an electronic aid may also go a long way toward clearing up the tinnitus or making it less noticeable. Additionally, while tinnitus maskers are available as stand-alone devices, they can also be incorporated in many hearing aids.

How Hearing Aids Work

Defined in the simplest manner, a hearing aid consists of three main parts:

1. A *microphone* which captures sound, translating its air vibrations into variations in electrical current.

2. An *amplifying stage* where these variations in electrical current are magnified many times (the degree of amplification being selected by the user through a volume control) to produce an output signal that is considerably greater than the original input received from the microphone.

3. An *earphone* (essentially a miniature loudspeaker) in which the amplified electrical variations are once again turned into air vibrations, these being directed via the external ear canal at the ear drum.

Additionally, there is a small battery that powers the whole system.

Types of Hearing Aids

According to the National Institute of Deafness and Other Communication Disorders (NIDCD), there are four basic types of hearing aids for people suffering from sensorineural hearing loss:

⬦ **In-The-Ear (ITE)** hearing aids, which fit completely in the outer ear and are used for mild to severe hearing loss. ITEs can accommodate mechanisms like a telecoil which improves sound transmissions during telephone calls. But their small size can lead to adjustment problems or feedback and they can be damaged by earwax or ear drainage.

◇ **Behind-The-Ear (BTE)** hearing aids are worn, as the name implies, behind the ear and connected to a plastic ear mold that fits inside the outer ear. The components are held behind the ear. These aids are used for people with mild to profound hearing loss. Poorly fitting BTE ear molds can lead to problems with feedback.

◇ **Canal Aids** fit into the ear canal and are available in two sizes. In-The-Canal (ITC) aids are customized to fit the size and shape of the ear canal. Completely-In-Canal (CIC) aids are largely concealed in the ear canal. Both are used for mild to moderate cases of hearing loss. Due to their small size both can be difficult to remove or adjust.

◇ **Body Aids** are used in cases of extreme hearing loss or when other types of aids cannot be used. They are attached to a belt or pocket and connected to the ear by a wire. Because of their large size, they can incorporate many signal processing options.

Types of Circuitry or Electronics

The inside mechanisms of hearing aids vary among the types of circuitry or electronics used:

◇ **Analog/Adjustable.** A laboratory builds the aid to meet the specifications you need as outlined by the audiologist. This type of circuitry is generally the least expensive.

◇ **Analog/Programmable.** The audiologist uses a computer to program your hearing aid. As the circuitry of this type of aid can accommodate more than one program or setting, the wearer can change the program in different listening environments with a remote control devise.

◇ **Digital/Programmable.** Digital aids use a microphone, receiver, battery and computer chip and provides the most flexibility for the audiologist to adjust the hearing aid to your needs. But this is also the most expensive option.

No matter what their configuration may be, hearing aids all work on the same principle: they amplify ambient sounds, making them loud enough to be picked by the deficient hearing. However useful these aids can be, they do have their limitations and will not always work as well as might be hoped. Here are some of the main factors that affect just how effective a hearing aid will be:

◊ Hearing aids are most likely to be of considerable help when the hearing loss lies mainly in frequencies between 100 and 4,000 Hz, as the instruments generally produce little or no amplification outside that band. However, this range isn't as restricted as it appears at first glance because it covers the frequencies used by normal speech, which are (quite naturally) the sounds that people with impaired hearing most want to be enabled to hear more clearly. Additionally, modern hearing aids also allow for the selective amplification of specific frequencies within that range, providing more volume to those frequencies where the hearing loss is greatest.

◊ While modern-day electronics can create extreme amplifications, too high an output volume from a hearing aid can cause further damage to what hearing is left. For most people the problem won't arise because a moderate degree of amplification is sufficient. Generally, hearing aids are most likely to provide maximum benefit when the loss is such that a gain of up to around 40 decibels is adequate. Should much greater amplification be needed, there is always a danger that this in itself may eventually lead to further hearing loss.

⬥ The greater the amplification needed, the greater the likelihood that the aid itself will become a source of noise. There are two ways in which this can happen. First of all, all amplifiers produce a certain amount of background noise. Usually this noise is so faint that it isn't noticed. But as you turn up the volume, the noise is also increased. What's more, the signal-to-noise ratio may worsen appreciably at high gain levels—"signal" denoting the sounds you want to hear. Secondly, the louder the output through the earphone, the more likely that some of this may also be picked up the microphone, resulting in feedback. Feedback means that the sound being output is also being fed back to the input, creating an endless loop of distorted sounds that gets louder and louder.

The Federal Trade Commission (FTC) is responsible for monitoring the business practices of hearing-aid dispensers and vendors (website: www.ftc.com; tel: 877-FTC-HELP). Here are a few points the FTC recommends that you keep in mind before buying a hearing aid:

⬥ Make sure the supplier is reputable and that the dispenser is licensed or certified by the state in which you live. You can check out prospective dispensers with your local better business bureau, consumer protection agency or state attorney general's office. It's also a really good idea to ask family and friends for referrals. Never feel pressured into buying a hearing aid. If you are not completely comfortable with the supplier, ask for more information or get a second opinion.

◊ Even when properly prescribed and fitted, hearing aids don't always work as well as might be expected. Most states recommend or require a minimum 30-day free trial period. You might be charged a "service fee" if you return the hearing aid during that time; this can range from five to 20% of the purchase price. Keep a lookout for manufacturers who allow returns within 90 days of purchase at no charge.

◊ It's not wise to buy hearing aids from door-to-door salesmen. If you do, the law allows you to cancel any sale of more than $25 within three business days—*if* the sale took place anywhere that is not the salesman's regular place of business.

◊ Some states don't allow hearing aids to be sold through the mail because it's hard to get a proper fit. However, if your state does allow mail-order sales, federal law requires that the company selling the devises ship your hearing aid when promised and give you a full refund if you decide to cancel your purchase.

◊ Read the hearing-aid purchase agreement or contract. It should include all terms of the transaction, including a clear explanation of all verbal promises. Check to see if the manufacturer or dispenser holds the warranty. In some cases, a manufacturer will not honor a warranty unless is the hearing aid was purchased from an authorized seller. Also check to see what services are provided free of charge, the length of time they will be provided, and whether you will receive a "loaner" if the hearing aid ever needs repair.

The Food and Drug Administration (FDA) enforces regulations covering the manufacture and sale of hearing aids. They say that the following conditions must be met by all dispensers of hearing aids:

◊ Dispensers must get a written statement from the patient, signed by a licensed physician and dated within the past six months, stating that the patient has undergone a physical exam and has been cleared for the fitting of a hearing aid.

◊ Anyone over the age of 18 can sign of waiver for the exam, but the dispenser must not encourage them to do this and must advise them that this is not in their best interest.

◊ If the patient has not yet seen a doctor for their hearing difficulties, the vendor must advise them to do so.

◊ Every hearing aid must come with an instructional booklet that describes its operation, use and care, as well a list of companies that provide repair and maintenance.

Just how much relief from tinnitus may be provided by a hearing aid varies greatly. But it's presumed that some improvement may follow for a quarter or even more of people whose tinnitus is accompanied by marked hearing loss. It's worth pointing out any improvement in tinnitus won't always be immediately noticeable. It takes time to get used to a hearing aid and learn how to use it for the best tinnitus-reducing effect.

Tinnitus Maskers

The basic principle of tinnitus masking is a simple one: if you're bothered by a sound but can't eliminate it, then the presence of another sound may counteract or "camouflage" the first one so that the obnoxious sound troubles you less, if at all.

All of us mask sounds—if we didn't, our lives would be quite intolerable because our brains would be assailed constantly by a barrage of all kinds of noises, most of which would be of no importance to us but which nevertheless would have to be recorded and analyzed. Were some kind of automatic filtering not applied by the brain to incoming sound data, the sheer magnitude of this information would soon lead to a sensory overload. However, the brain's ability to discriminate between important sounds and those which aren't allows us to concentrate upon those that matter while more or less ignoring the rest.

Much of this filtering activity operates automatically, probably as the result of countless generations of evolutionary change. But the brain can also quite rapidly adapt this process to meet specific circumstances. For example, someone living near a railway line may soon become blissfully unaware of trains roaring by—the brain learns to pay little or no attention to these sounds, recognizing them as being unimportant at the time. The brain's sound-filtering ability is put to good effect in tinnitus masking, a technique based on the artificial creation of an *additional* sound aimed at reducing the impact of tinnitus noises.

The masking device produces a sound, which although perhaps louder than the tinnitus, is of a type that the brain finds easier to ignore. Although all kinds of noises can result from tinnitus, the most common ones are fairly high-pitched tones, which are often exceptionally unpleasant and particularly difficult to ignore. On the other hand, a sound like the gentle gurgling of a fountain is a lot easier to ignore and, even when consciously perceived, a great deal more pleasant than tinnitus. In practice, what this means is that when someone is receiving an artificially created sound, as he or she learns to ignore this, so the underlying tinnitus may no longer be perceived as clearly as before.

The masking principle can be utilized in several ways, the most common ones including:

⬦ **Electronic Devices Worn In or Behind the Ear.** Looking essentially like hearing aids, these devices can form part of (or be an addition to) a normal hearing aid. Depending upon the actual device, the wearer may have a great deal of control in choosing or altering the masking sound, altering its volume and fundamental pitch, as well as what frequencies it will be at its loudest. The audiometry can provide clues as to what kind of masking sound is most likely to be helpful in a given case, but the user may still have to experiment quite a bit until the optimum relief is obtained. While the masker may be effective in "blanking out" the tinnitus noises, the user is initially very aware of the masking

109

sound and it may be several weeks or longer before the masker can be ignored.

◇ **Radios, CD Players, etc**. Many tinnitus sufferers have found that merely having a radio or CD playing at low volume can be an effective tinnitus masker. Generally, this works best if the external sounds are fairly monotonous, like so-called "easy listening" music. It can also be useful to experiment with the tone controls (or graphic equalizer) of the amplifier by selecting settings that heighten one or more frequencies in the treble while cutting down the bass. This usually makes for more effective masking. In some cases, the greatest masking effect is produced by deliberately not tuning your radio to a station. The resultant hissing, crackling sound—a mixture of noises at various frequencies—is often an excellent masker.

◇ **Special Tinnitus Masking Audio Tapes.** A number of tapes containing sounds designed to work particularly well for a wide cross-section of tinnitus sufferers have been recorded by experts.

◇ **Wide Band Noise Generators.** An advanced form of masker that contains all frequencies and gently stimulates all nerves in subconscious networks, allowing them to be reset to the point that the tinnitus signals can no longer be detected. They also reduce the contrast between tinnitus noise and total silence.

Apart from these ways of masking tinnitus, you can also experiment yourself with a variety of sounds. Some of the sounds that tinnitus sufferers report as effective maskers are quite surprising, including such things as washing machines and the chirping of caged birds. In fact, just about any sound in existence has been credited by one tinnitus sufferer or another as being of help in their case.

Masking, of course, will not work for everyone. One quick way of establishing whether masking is likely to be of help to you is this simple test:

⬦ Stand reasonably close to a sink and turn on one of the taps, letting the water run freely.

⬦ Ask yourself whether the sound of the running water completely obscures your tinnitus? If the water masks the tinnitus, then there's every chance that a masker will do the same. Should your tinnitus still remain clearly audible above the sound of the water, then the chances are slimmer that a masker will make a great deal of difference.

111

This test, of course, provides only a broad indication. Regardless of outcome, it's still worth investigating whether some other sort of masking sound will be effective.

Summing Things Up

While masking works by providing a more easily ignored or more pleasant sound than tinnitus, another way of minimizing the impact of the disorder is reducing how strongly you react to (or are affected by) the noises you hear. In the next chapter, we will look at different ways of doing exactly that.

CHAPTER 8

Psychological Aspects of Tinnitus

While medical treatments, hearing aids and masking devices—plus the avoidance of things that make the disorder worse—can bring major relief in many cases of tinnitus, it remains a sad fact that these approaches don't work for everyone. For some, relief may often be found in one or more psychological techniques.

Such approaches will leave the physical problem (which manifests itself as tinnitus) totally unchanged. But what *can* be altered is how much the noises affect you and your ability to ignore them. Psychology, of course, is the science concerned with human behavior and this very broad classification encompasses a large number of different schools of thought, some of these based on what appears to be conflicting theories and methods. Just how useful psychological approaches are in battling tinnitus will vary considerably from patient to patient, but experts generally agree upon the following key points:

◊ While not all tinnitus is directly related to stress, anxiety or depression, the extent to which patients will react to (and be affected by) their disorder is often greatly influenced by their state of mind.

◊ An undue level of stress for lengthy periods is often the first stepping stone that leads to other psychological difficulties later. Any chronic disorder, especially one whose symptoms are as difficult to ignore as tinnitus, will almost certainly be a source of considerable additional stress.

◊ While they are separate disorders, there are close links between anxiety and depression, one frequently preceding the other. The symptoms of almost any ailment (including tinnitus) often appear to be at their worst when the patient is also in an anxious or depressed state.

◊ It's not uncommon for there to be a vicious cycle in which the tinnitus creates anxiety or other psychological problems;

the heightened anxiety then making the tinnitus seems worse than it really is. This, in turn, often leads to further and possibly greater anxiety. If this cycle can't be broken by curing the tinnitus, then its overall harmful effect may be greatly diminished by reducing the anxiety level.

This means that anything which addresses the problem of undue stress is likely to pay rich dividends in tinnitus in two quite separate ways:

1. The less stressed you feel, the less bothered you're likely to be by tinnitus.

2. Because the tinnitus will bother you less, the disorder will itself become a lesser source of stress.

What Exactly is Stress?

In a medical context, stress is normally defined as any factor that threatens the health of the body or has an adverse effect on its functioning. However, psychologists generally prefer a different definition that states: "Stress is the non-specific response of the body to any demand." The key part of this last definition, of course, is the phrase "non-specific," which identifies a response that isn't necessary or useful in dealing with the problem at hand. For example, getting agitated about your tinnitus isn't going to help you cope any better with its symptoms.

There are many different kinds of tests and psychological inventories aimed at determining whether someone is unduly stressed, but these are likely to be rather superfluous in the case of someone afflicted with severe tinnitus. Generally, it can be safely assumed that anyone with severe tinnitus is subject to high stress, with the cumulative effect of that stress possibly leading to anxiety.

While there are many ways to reduce stress and/or anxiety, the techniques used most commonly when dealing with tinnitus are either drug treatments, relaxation techniques, or a combination of both.

Drug Treatments to Relieve Stress

Whether or not you should be prescribed drugs to relieve stress associated with tinnitus is a question for your doctor. But the way you choose to present your problems may well affect his or her decision. Drugs that may be prescribed in these circumstances include:

⬥ **Benzodiazepines.** These drugs (*lorazepam* and *diazepam* are probably the best known and most widely prescribed) were first introduced more than 30 years ago and are still considered to be a first line of defense against anxiety symptoms. Although the Committee on Safety of Medicines has recommended that benzodiazepines be considered inappropriate for the treatment of short-term "mild" anxiety, this recommendation is not observed by many doctors.

While these drugs can be highly effective, their use does entail a high risk of dependence. There are also some possible side effects including drowsiness, headaches and vertigo.

◊ **MAOIs.** The initials stand for "monoamine oxidase inhibitors." Used to treat both anxiety and depression, these drugs are particularly effective in treating high levels of stress that culminate in so-called "panic attacks." Great caution, however, must be exercised with these medications because they can interact dangerously with some common foods as well as with other drugs. For this reason, their use is usually avoided when safer preparations may be equally suitable.

◊ **Antidepressants.** Despite their name, these can be more effective in the treatment of anxiety than drugs meant specifically for that purpose, and they carry a much lower risk of dependency. On the

117

other hand, antidepressants can be slow in producing results and patients may not persevere long enough to gain worthwhile benefits. Additionally, these drugs have been known to create side effects including apprehension, insomnia and irritability. Antidepressants must be used very cautiously in treating tinnitus because they can make the problem worse.

For additional information about some of these drugs, also see the sections headed "Drug Treatments for Tinnitus" at the end of Chapter 5 and "Drugs That May Worsen Matters" in Chapter 6.

Relaxation Techniques

While drugs may bring quite rapid relief from stress and anxiety, they merely reduce the symptoms that an emotional overload can create. As useful as this can be to get someone over a bad patch, it's not an ideal long-term solution. On the other hand, relaxation techniques can be equally effective in combating stress and anxiety—without any risk of side effects or harmful dependence.

There are many different kinds of relaxation methods, but the ones used most commonly to relieve anxiety are based on the principle that mental relaxation will come as a by-product of attaining physical relaxation. This concept of using the body to relax the mind (or vice versa) is one whose validity has been proven beyond doubt by countless experimental studies.

For more information about relaxation techniques:

◊ Ask your family doctor. Many of the more enlightened practices nowadays operate special classes in relaxation techniques.

◊ Alternatively, your doctor may refer you to the nearest hospital or community center where relaxation techniques are taught, either on a one-to-one basis or in group sessions.

◊ Check with your local adult education institute. Many of these run relaxation classes.

◊ Should none of these approaches yield results, you'll almost certainly find several "do-it-yourself books" on the subject at your local library or bookstore.

Other Psychologically-Based Approaches

The following stress-reduction techniques are usually only available to patients attending special tinnitus clinics attached to the ear, nose and throat departments of larger hospitals. Generally, only patients with severe tinnitus aggravated by stress and/or anxiety will be candidates for these treatments, which are often part of research programs.

◊ **Biofeedback training**. This technique works by providing the subject with immediate information about a bodily function that normally operates unconsciously. During a biofeedback training session, the patient is connected to a monitor measuring unconscious body activities such as blood pressure, pulse rate, body temperature and muscle tension. The monitoring equipment feeds information about changes in the levels of these activities to the patient, either through flashing lights, a needle moving on a dial, or altering tone pitch. With practice, the patient learns how to exercise conscious control over the unconscious function being monitored. In tinnitus, the technique has been used with some success to reduce muscular tension, promoting overall relaxation, which leads to lessened perception of the noises. Most commonly, biofeedback is used in conjunction with normal deep-relaxation techniques.

◊ **Cognitive-behavioral therapy**. Based on the concept that the way in which we perceive our environment and ourselves influences our emotions and behavior, cognitive-behavioral therapy seeks to alter these perceptions into more positive ones. For example, someone suffering from anxiety or depression may believe that undesirable events are the result of a failing on his or her part. The therapist will attempt to identify negative attitudes and irrational beliefs, leading the patient to see problems more positively and optimistically, thereby automatically easing anxiety or emotional distress associated with them. If a patient can be brought to see his problem as less troublesome, then it often follows that its symptoms will bother him less.

⋄ **Tinnitus Retraining Therapy**. TRT is designed to retrain the brain to ignore the tinnitus through a combination of counseling (teaching, demystifying, reevaluation, desensitization) and masking or the use of a wide-band noise generator. Over time, some patients learn to ignore the tinnitus. But this treatment option takes time—the recommended course of treatment can be more than a year. This process is also called *habituation* of reaction. One of the foremost advocates of this treatment, Dr. Pawel Jasterboff, says that repetitive exposure to subconscious sound can change reflexive reactions and extinguish undesired responses.

Psychological approaches also often play a large part in many of the alternative or complementary medicine treatments discussed in the next chapter.

CHAPTER 9

Alternative Medicine Treatments

Because there is often little that conventional medicine can do for tinnitus, it's not surprising that many sufferers have sought help from practitioners of so-called "alternative" or "complementary" therapies. While it's unlikely these therapies will be able to address the cause of the tinnitus or cure it, they can be of great assistance in altering the patient's perception of the problem and so make it easier to bear.

Generally, alternative therapies emphasize a patient's overall well-being instead of concentrating solely on a given ailment. This sort of approach—which normally uses a wide variety of methods to alleviate mental and/or emotional stress—can work very well for some tinnitus sufferers and pay rich dividends in enhanced quality of life.

The reasons why someone afflicted by a chronic health problem seeks help from practitioners of alternative forms of medicine are often highly individual. But the main ones, according to a recent survey, include:

⋄ If there is no definite, clear-cut cause for a disorder and its existence may be linked to emotional state, patients may conclude that alternative treatments (with their emphasis on the "whole person") may bring improvements where conventional medicine failed to do so.

⋄ Many alternative therapies have a good track record in helping people to cope better with all sorts of ongoing health problems, especially those which are chronic or where the severity of the symptoms is affected by numerous seemingly unconnected factors.

⋄ Alternative therapies—particularly those whose philosophy stresses the power of "mind over matter"—can help a patient comply with some of the health recommendations suggested by their doctor. For example, smoking has been implicated in worsening, if not outright causing, tinnitus. While it is therefore sensible to give up the habit, it's not always such an easy thing to do. The support provided by some alternative therapies can, however, ease the pangs of withdrawal.

While the vast majority of alternative practitioners are highly trained and totally ethical, there is a "fringe element" whose standards are less than adequate. Here are some suggestions that can help you select a reputable alternative practitioner:

◊ Ensure that you pick a fully accredited member of a professional body whose standing is recognized.

◊ Although medical doctors aren't meant to recommend alternative practitioners, you may discover that your own family doctor is prepared to do just that—although you may have to "read between the lines" of what he or she is recommending. Nowadays, most general practitioners are much more open-minded about the benefits that alternative therapies can bring and accepting that disciplines like hypnosis or acu-

> puncture can help some people control stress levels.

> ◇ Word-of-mouth recommendations are also extremely useful. Personal endorsements from people whose judgment you respect can be a good guide.

No matter how carefully you've chosen your alternative practitioner, it's always a good idea to also consult your doctor beforehand and tell them what you have in mind. Later on, you may also wish to check the safety aspects of any alternative treatments with your own doctor.

A great resource on alternative medicine is the National Center for Complementary and Alternative Medicine (NCCAM). A component of the National Institutes of Health, it provides a wealth of information about health care outside the realm of conventional medicine as practiced in the United States. However, they do not provide medical advice or referrals to practitioners.

The National Center for Complementary and Alternative Medicine
PO Box 7923, Gaithersburg, MD 20898
Tel: 888-644-6226 or 301-519-3153
   or TTY 866-464-3615
Fax: 866-464-3616
Website: www.nccam.nih.gov
Email: info@nccam.nih.gov

While there are dozens (if not hundreds) of different alternative therapies to choose from, some seem to be more helpful than others in dealing with tinnitus, according to reports from patients. Here are brief details of the ones that are most likely to deserve consideration:

Homeopathy

Probably the most generally accepted form of alternative medicine, homeopathy is a treatment system devised in the late 1700s by Samuel Hahnemann. Homeopathy is based on two essential and intertwined principles—the cure for an ailment is often found in whatever brought it on in the first instance; and small dosages of medication are usually more effective than larger ones. Like many alternative practitioners, homeopaths also believe that symptoms are signs produced by the body's own attempts to ward off or cure infection or disease.

Homeopathic practitioners maintain that the human body has an inbuilt capability to cope with and recover from most illnesses and that the healer's primary job is to strengthen the patient's innate ability to heal oneself. To aid and stimulate the body's natural mechanisms to accomplish that task, treatment is usually administered as extremely small doses of various medications, usually prepared from natural substances and originating from a wide variety of herbal, animal, mineral and metallic sources.

The guiding principle of "minimal dose" often leads to remedies that are so diluted that none of the original healing ingredient can still be detected in the final mixture or solution. Naturally, this has led skeptics to question how a medicine can have a therapeutic effect if there is nothing— or at best, very little—left of the original "healing" substance? Homeopaths are the first to admit that they don't know why these extremely diluted remedies should have any effect, but point with pride to the vast mountain of clinical evidence that appears to prove beyond any shadow of doubt that they often do.

Because homeopathic remedies are so diluted, you don't need a prescription to buy them and you can obtain them across the counter in many pharmacies and health stores. While, theoretically, this makes it possible for a patient to prescribe his own medication, practitioners point out that it takes a great deal of skill and experience to choose the correct remedy for a given situation because diagnostic procedure takes into account not only the nature of the ailment but also the patient as whole. As a result, different remedies may be prescribed for different forms of the same problem.

For example, if you look up tinnitus in *The Prescriber* (a kind of mini-bible of the main homeopathic preparations) you'll discover that suggested treatments depends a number of factors including the nature of the sounds heard, whether the condition is chronic or not, and whether there is observable deafness. Additionally, treatments should be matched to other aspects of the patient's health. With so many possible permutations, choosing the right remedy and dosage is obviously something that requires an expert. You can get more information about homeopathy from:

National Center for Homeopathy
801 N. Fairfax Street, Suite 306 Alexandria,
    Virginia 22314
Tel: 877-624-0613 or 703-548-7790
Fax: (703) 548-7792
Website: www.homeopathic.org
Email: info@homeopathic.org

North American Society of Homeopaths
1122 East Pike Street, #1122, Seattle,
    Washington 98122
Tel: 206-720-7000
Fax: 208-248-1942
Website: www.homeopathy.org
Email: nashinfo@aol.com

Acupuncture and Acupressure

One of the most revered of the ancient Asian medical arts, acupuncture was first widely practiced in China more than 2,000 years ago. The therapy works by using fine needles (or other similar objects) to stimulate specific points on the body and so create changes in other parts of it. One of the aims of this system is to "rebalance" forces to improve health.

Acupuncturists believe in the Chinese philosophy that within all of us dwells a basic life force (*chi*) composed of two energy flows—a positive one called "yin" and a negative one called "yang." These energy flows course throughout the body along channels known as "meridians." Disease and pain are the result of an imbalance or interruption in their normal flow.

Although acupuncture has become one of the better established and widely accepted forms of alternative medicine in the Western world and has a long record of being effective in treating a wide range of disorders, there is a great deal of doubt about whether it can truly make much of a difference in tinnitus. There is little or no objective evidence to demonstrate that acupuncture can have an affect. Despite that, there is no question that many tinnitus sufferers most emphatically believe that acupuncture has helped them. However, this claim is dismissed by most medical researchers who attribute any perceived improvement to a placebo effect.

Acupressure works broadly on the same principles—and can provide similar benefits—as acupuncture.

In acupressure, the various pressure points on the body are massaged by the practitioner's finger or thumb instead of being stimulated by the introduction of needles. One big advantage of this method is that it is often possible for patients to be taught how to perform this massage for themselves and so be able to continue their treatment on their own, using acupressure as often as required.

Most acupuncturists also offer acupressure, not because it's necessarily any better, but rather because some people just cannot face the idea of having needles stuck into them. Because it's absolutely essential that the needles used in acupuncture be sterile, it's always best to consult a fully qualified practitioner. Many states have their own acupuncturist association. Contact details for most of them can be obtained from:

American Association of Oriental Medicine
5530 Wisconsin Avenue, #1210, Chevy Chase, MD 20815
Tel: 301-941-1064 or 888-500-7999
Fax: 301-986-9313
Website: www.aaom.org
Email:info@aaom.org

Hypnosis and Hypnotherapy

Of all the alternative therapies used to minimize the effects of tinnitus, hypnosis and hypnotherapy are some of the most successful. The effects of these approaches, which are used both by doctors and alternative practitioners, are well documented and have rendered excellent results in cases where sufferers have failed to respond to other treatments. Because there is a great deal of difference between hypnosis practitioners, it's particularly important that you choose your hypnotherapist with great care.

Both hypnosis and hypnotherapy rely essentially on the power of suggestion, whether this suggestion comes from the therapist or from the patient himself. In fact, there is a school of thought that no one is ever hypnotized by someone else because the subjects are actually hypnotizing themselves, with the hypnotist merely providing a conduit for this self-hypnosis. Be that as it may, one extremely valuable aspect of hypnosis is that most patients can be successfully taught to hypnotize themselves and they can then use the technique on their own, whenever needed, to further reinforce suggestions received during previous sessions.

A good deal of research has gone into the effectiveness of hypnosis in tinnitus. Although there are some variations in the findings of different studies, the general conclusion is that hypnosis brings worthwhile benefits for many tinnitus sufferers. The results show that the technique is particularly suitable for reducing the effects of tinnitus exacerbated by stress or worry. However, experts agree that hypnosis doesn't actually reduce the tinnitus itself, but makes it appear better because the patient's reaction to his or her tinnitus is modified, either by making them less aware of the noises or increasing their level of tolerance to them.

Not everyone is a suitable candidate for hypnosis and there is considerable variation in the degree to which people respond to the technique. Some fall almost immediately into a deep trance-like state at the first suggestion, while others totally fail to respond. Post-hypnotic suggestions can work extremely well even if the subject's trance is so minimal that they remain totally unaware that they are (or have been) in a hypnotic state.

One way of trying out hypnosis at little cost and with minimal risk is by buying a self-hypnosis tape. While not geared specifically to tinnitus, many of these tapes can be adapted by the user so that the suggestions they contain become directly relevant to the problem. Incidentally, many hypnotists will provide patients with an individualized tape they can use at home.

Just how successful "taped" hypnosis can be was demonstrated in a study of 32 tinnitus patients. Each initially received a one-hour session with a therapist, during which post-hypnotic suggestions were implanted and a tape made containing suggestions that the tinnitus noises were gradually becoming less troublesome. For the next month, the patients were told to listen to the tape once every day at home. At the end of the study, 22 patients (just over a third) reported that they were "considerably" less troubled by their tinnitus.

Important: Although many hypnotherapists are medically qualified doctors, many others are not. You have to decide for yourself whether you want your hypnotherapist to also be a doctor. If you believe that hypnosis could help you, discuss this option with your doctor. Alternatively, you can get more information from:

The American Board of Hypnotherapy
2002 E. McFadden Ave., #100, Santa Ana
   CA 92705
Tel: 714-245-9340 Toll free: 800-872-9996
Fax: 714-245-9881
Website: www.hypnosis.com/abh/abh
Email: laih@hypnosis.com

International Medical and Dental
   Hypnotherapy Association *(IMDHA)*
4110 Edgeland, #800, Royal Oak, MI
   48073-2285
Tel: 248-549-5594 Toll free: 800-257-5467
Website: www.infinityinst.com

Yoga

Yoga is a very ancient discipline originally developed on the Indian subcontinent. There are many different forms of yoga, but these can be divided into two main categories:

1) Physical exercises—primarily stretching the limbs, back and neck—that promote strength and flexibility as well as emphasizing breath control.

2) A meditation discipline that aims to help the subject achieve a state of peace and harmony in the inner self through mental control and relaxation.

Both of these aspects of yoga are meant to work together to bring about a "healthy mind in a healthy body." However, the physical exercises can be practiced on their own. Yoga has a proven record as being extremely effective in reducing stress levels and is therefore of likely benefit to many tinnitus sufferers. For those who can spare the considerable time involved in learning them, the meditation techniques have shown to help reduce the effects of tinnitus.

While nearly all yoga exercises are considered to be safe for a moderately fit person, there are nevertheless some that create great strain on the back and abdomen and as such should be approached with caution and only under the guidance of a competent teacher. Glaucoma sufferers are also advised to avoid any exercises involving holding an upside-down position for any length of time. For these reasons, all but the very simplest of yoga exercises should only be undertaken under proper supervision. It's also a good idea to check beforehand with your doctor whether he or she thinks yoga is a good idea in the circumstances of your particular case.

You can get more information from:

> ***American Yoga Association***
> P.O. Box 19986, Sarasota, FL 34276
> Tel: 941-927-4977
> Fax 941-921-9844
> Website: www.americanyogaassociation.org
> Email: info@americanyogaassociation.org

The following Website also provides some useful links to yoga-related sites:

> www.yogadirectory.com/
> Reference_and_Resources/Associations/

Music Therapy

Music therapy is also used for stress and anxiety reduction, as well as pain management and to effect positive mood changes. It's currently being used around the world to help people with hearing impairments. But to-date, only a few clinics are concentrating on using music therapy to treat tinnitus. In Germany, psychotherapist Martin Kusatz has developed a form of therapy which comprises a blend of counseling, music therapy sessions, movement therapy and medical consultations. After a six-month test of 700 tinnitus sufferers, 3.2—said they no longer had tinnitus, 30.8% reported a reduction in the sounds of tinnitus and about two thirds of the test patients said their tinnitus was less troubling.

Other Alternative Therapies

Some of the disciplines described above are so well established they are often seen as an adjunct to conventional treatment rather than an alternative to it. There are, however, several other complementary therapies that have been found helpful by at least some tinnitus sufferers. Here are details of some other alternative therapies you may wish to consider.

Naturopathy. Also known as "naturopathic medicine," this is broadly-based system that combines a wide variety of natural therapeutic and healing techniques under a virtually all-encompassing umbrella. Naturopathy can perhaps be best described as a mixture of traditional folk wisdom and modern medicine. The underlying principle of this therapy is that the root-cause of all disease is the accumulation of waste products and toxins in the human body, usually the result of a "deficient" life style.

Like many alternative practitioners, naturopaths also subscribe to the view that our bodies have the wisdom and power to heal themselves, providing that we enhance rather than interfere with this natural process. As far as treatments are concerned, naturopathy relies heavily on herbal preparations and diet management techniques. Treatments offered by a naturopath may include the following: physiotherapy (based on water), ultrasound, heat and/or cold, yoga and breathing exercises, biofeedback techniques, and corrective nutrition.

A key aspect of the naturopathic approach is that it relies very heavily upon the practitioner and the patient discussing and agreeing upon what therapies to use. It also emphasizes the promotion of psychological health and the benefits of stress reduction. Although individual patients' experiences vary, many have said it helps them cope better with tinnitus.

You can get more information from:

The American Association of Naturopathic Physicians
3201 New Mexico Avenue, NW # 350,
    Washington, DC 20016
Tel: 202-895-1392 Toll free: 866-538-2267
Fax: 202-274-1992

Website: www.naturopathic.org
Email: member.services@Naturopathic.org

Herbalism. Almost certainly the most ancient of all medical systems, herbalism (also called herbal medicine) uses plants and their by-products to prevent and treat disease. In this context, it needs to be noted that there is a difference between what the word "herb" means to a botanist (any plant that doesn't have woody fibers and no persistent parts above the ground) and to a herbalist (any plant credited with having medicinal value). Accordingly, herbal medicine encompasses the use of any plant, as well as any part of it, including the leaf, stem, seed, root, bark or flower.

Most modern herbalists practice their discipline in keeping with the age-old tradition which decrees that medicines are not just used to treat disease, but are also a way to return the body's balance to its normal state (disease or pain being considered "abnormal"). Naturally, this means that a given disorder may not always be treated by the same herbal preparation. Deciding on the right treatment in a given case is influenced by a number of factors including the patient's general health, disposition and even personality.

Despite this highly individualistic approach to diagnosis and treatment, there are many different "pharmacopoeias" (listings of specific remedies linked to conditions). Some of these have origins dating back as many as 6,000 years ago, when the Chinese first started classifying and cataloguing herbal cures.

Herbal remedies are formulated in a wide variety of forms, the main ones being teas, potions, juices, extracts, bath additives, salves, lotions and ointments.

While there is a great deal to be said in favor of herbalism, a note of caution needs to be sounded. Many herbal remedies are just as powerful—and potentially just as toxic if not prescribed or administered correctly—as modern-day drugs. This naturally means that these preparations must be handled with extreme care as they can otherwise produce harmful side effects. It is therefore absolutely essential that herbal remedies be prescribed by and used under the supervision of a suitably qualified medical herbalist.

You can get more information from:

> ***American Herbalists Guild***
> 1931 Gaddis Road, Canton, GA 30115
> Tel: 770-751-6021 Fax: 770-751-7472
> Website: www.americanherbalistsguild.com
> Email: ahgoffice@earthlink.net

Aromatherapy. Similar to the field of herbalism, although more narrow, aromatherapy uses "essential oils" derived or extracted from wild or cultivated plants, herbs, fruits and trees, to restore the body's natural functions and rhythms. The essences are prepared so that they can be used in many different ways, but most commonly as compresses, bath additives, inhalants or massaging lubricants.

Although there is little conventional medical research to support their claims, aromatherapists maintain that treatments can be useful in controlling tinnitus by reducing anxiety, stress and tension. Bear in mind, however, that some of the oils used in aromatherapy can be poisonous if used other than in the very smallest quantities. It's therefore vital that this therapy be administered only by a suitably qualified practitioner.

You can get more information from:

> *The National Association for Holistic Aromatherapy*
> 4509 Interlake Ave N., #233,Seattle, WA 98103-6773
> Tel: 888-ASK-NAHA or 206-547-2164
> Fax: 206-547-2680
> Website: www.naha.org
> Email: info@naha.org

Additionally, this website provides an easy-to-understand overview of the benefits of aromatherapy: www.aworldofaromatherapy.com

Osteopathy. Developed in 1874 by Andrew Taylor Still, osteopathy has been found to be very effective in the relief of many stress-induced ailments and as such can have a role to play in reducing the reaction to tinnitus in some instances with treatments such as cranial sacral therapy. Based upon the underlying principle that "structure governs function," osteopathy relies mainly on manipulative techniques that are primarily applied to the back and the neck.

This alternative approach has gained great acceptance from the medical profession as a whole. Because of this level of recognition, your doctor may be able to suggest a good local practitioner. Once again, however, a note of caution is in order: it has been found in some instances that spinal manipulation can actually make tinnitus worse. It's vital that your osteopath fully understands tinnitus and is aware of what kind of manipulation could lead to problems. Always remember that while osteopathy can be helpful, it's also a potentially dangerous form of treatment which (if administered incorrectly) can end up doing more harm than good. It is essential that you find a reputable and skillful therapist.

You can get more information from:

American Osteopathic Association
142 East Ontario Street, Chicago, IL 60611
Tel: 312-202-8000

Toll free: 800-621-1773
Fax: 312-202-8200
Website: www.aoa-net.org
Email:info@aoa-net.org.

Healing and "Fringe" Therapies

Because the success of alternative therapies often relies greatly upon the link between physical and mental well-being—a link whose importance is nowadays fully accepted by conventional modern medicine—it can be extremely difficult to gauge what can or cannot be helpful for at least some tinnitus sufferers. Even "fringe" disciplines have their staunch supporters who say that various methods have helped them "accept" their tinnitus and that this acceptance has made the condition less disabling. Here are brief details of the two most commonly encountered healing therapies:

Healing. There are many different kinds of so-called "healing" techniques including faith, psychic, spiritual and energy, as well as the laying on of hands.

Throughout the ages, healers have been given credit for "curing" or alleviating all sorts of ailments and diseases, including tinnitus. However, it needs to be stated that there is little objective medical evidence to substantiate most of these claims. Despite that, numerous studies have shown how strong the power of suggestion can be. Therefore, it must be accepted that merely being told "you can no longer hear the noises that trouble you" by someone in whom you have faith, can indeed bring about a positive reaction, even if only temporary.

Therapeutic Touch. Like many healers, practitioners of therapeutic touch use a laying on of hands technique. This approach depends upon "human energy transfer in the act of healing" and is intended for use by non-psychics.

Summing Things Up

Several alternative therapies have helped many people live more comfortably with tinnitus. However, the success rate of others is a good deal patchier. Perhaps the single most important question is one that you should ask yourself: Do you believe that one of these therapies can help you?

CHAPTER 10

Self-Help Tips

This section will focus on natural and alternative steps that you can take yourself in order to relieve tinnitus symptoms. But remember these measures are not intended as a substitute for professional health care advice. You should always check with your health-care provider before trying any of these self-help tips.

If you have any interest at all in natural and alternative therapies, you're not alone. Studies show that as many as one in two American adults use some form of alternative medicine. And according to the American Medical Association, over half of U.S. medical schools now offer courses on acupuncture, herbs and other forms of holistic treatment in response to increasing interest in alternative medicine by the American public.

The following natural and alternative self-help tips may offer the kind of relief you've been looking for but were unable to achieve through conventional Western medicine.

Yoga Exercises

Increasing circulation of blood to the head has been reported to alleviate tinnitus symptoms. The following yoga exercises may help:

◊ Sit in a comfortable position.

◊ Turn your head slowly to the right as far as it will comfortably go, keeping your chin tucked in. Hold this position for a few seconds. Then turn your head slowly to the left as far as it will comfortably go, once again keeping your chin tucked in. Hold this position for a few seconds.

◊ Repeat three times.

◊ Tilting your head forward, bring your chin towards your chest and hold for a few seconds. Then tilt your head backward (while keeping your chin tucked in) and return to the starting position.

◊ Repeat three times.

Acupressure

Massage the points (shown below) which relate to tinnitus problems for at least five minutes the first day, increasing to at least five minutes twice a day. With your thumb, apply vigorous (but not painful) pressure.

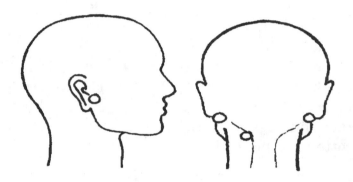

Relaxation Techniques

Relaxation techniques are of great value to many people especially in reducing stress, lowering blood pressure and improving functioning of the immune system.

Your eyes use up about one-quarter of the nervous energy consumed by your entire body says Dr. Edmund Jacobson of the University of Chicago. As a result, relaxing your eyes can relax your entire body. Try this simple method:

◇   Lean back and close your eyes.

◊ Silently say to your eyes "Let go...Stop frowning...Stop Straining...Let go."

◊ Repeat for at least one minute.

Herbal Ear Drops

An all-natural formula from Sweden has been reported to relieve the ringing and buzzing sounds of tinnitus. Called Bio Ear, the formula is made with aloe plus ginseng root, bitter orange, dandelion root, myrrh, saffron, senna leaves, camphor rhubarb root, zedoary root, carline thistle root and angelica root. The drops are applied to cotton and placed in the ears.

For more information on Bio Ear contact:

Penn Herb Company
Tel: 800-523-9971
Website: www.pennherb.com/pennherb/info/
scan56.html

Foot Reflexology

Reflexology is based on the belief that various organs, nerves and glands in your body are connected with certain "reflex areas" on the bottom of your feet. Each of the reflex areas of the feet relate to a specific part of the body. Massaging these areas is believed to send a surge of stimulation where needed to help clear out "congestion" and help restore normal functioning.

148

Reflexology techniques can be accomplished practically anyplace. No special equipment or training is needed. And reflexology can be done at home, at the office, in your car, or while watching television. The massage technique is simple to do, natural and safe.

⬦ Sit in a comfortable chair, sofa or on the floor.

⬦ Cross one of your legs over the other, resting the foot on the opposite knee as shown in the following diagram.

⬦ Massage the foot-reflex areas shown below that relate to the ears and the tinnitus condition. Massage for five minutes the first day and increase to at least five minutes twice a day.

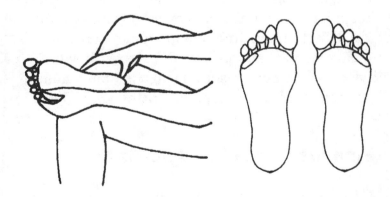

Foods that May Bring Relief

Getting insufficient amounts of specific nutrients in your diet may cause various medical and health problems, including tinnitus. A deficiency of the trace mineral manganese and the B vitamin choline may cause tinnitus symptoms, according to *Foods that Heal.*

The recommended daily allowance of manganese is 2.5 to 5 mg. Foods high in manganese include bananas, celery, cereals, green leafy vegetables, beans, nuts and whole grains. If you believe you may not be getting adequate amounts of this essential trace mineral, consider supplementing your diet.

The RDA for choline has not been established, but a level of about 500 mg per day is generally considered adequate for proper body functioning. Foods high in choline include fish, beans, organ meats, soybeans and brewer's yeast. If you believe you are not consuming an adequate amount of choline, consider supplementing your diet.

Tinnitus Caused by Anemia

Certain types of anemia can cause tinnitus symptoms. *Foods that Heal* reports that medical doctor Jonathan Wright has reversed tinnitus by supplementing the diet with vitamin B12 and iron.

Iron-deficiency anemia is caused by a shortage of the mineral iron required to produce hemoglobin. The shortage of iron can be caused by a variety of factors including a diet lacking in dark-green vegetables and organ meats, pregnancy and excessive menstrual flow.

The RDA for iron is between 10 and 18 mg. Foods high in iron include fish, lean meat, beans and whole grains. If you believe you are not getting sufficient amounts of iron in your diet consider supplements.

Pernicious anemia is caused by the body's inability to absorb vitamin B12 in amounts sufficient to produce normal quantities of red blood cells. This can be caused by an inflamed bowel, parasites or small intestine disorders. The RDA of vitamin B12 is 3 mcg. Foods high in vitamin B12 include beef, fish and dairy products. If you believe you are not getting adequate supplies of vitamin B12 consider supplementing your diet.

Hand Reflexology

Similar to foot reflexology, this technique is based on "reflex area" in the hands connected to specific organs in the body. Massaging these reflex areas is believed by proponents to send a surge of stimulation where needed in the body to help clear out "congestion" and restore normal functioning.

Like foot reflexology, hand reflexology can be done almost anywhere. No special devices or training is required.

It's important to remember when performing the hand reflexology exercises detailed below that your right hand specifically relates to your right ear, and likewise your left hand to your left ear. If you suffer tinnitus in only one ear, it may still be a good idea to work on both hands. This may help prevent future problems in the unaffected ear.

◊   Sit in a comfortable chair and relax.

◊   Following the following illustration, massage the reflex areas on each hand for about five minutes the first day. Starting the second day, massage for at least five minutes twice a day.

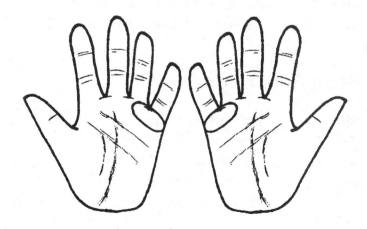

Ginkgo Biloba

Chinese herbalists have recommended ginkgo biloba as a valuable nutritional factor for more 2,000 years. *Pharmaceutical-grade ginkgo biloba extract (GBE)* has gone through no less than 40 clinical trials, the majority of which report that is the compound is indeed helpful for people with tinnitus. The evidence is so strong that the German Commission E, responsible for regulating and approving phytomedicinals in that country, formally endorses the use of ginkgo biloba for the treatment of tinnitus.

As of yet, it has not been scientifically established why ginkgo biloba brings relief from tinnitus. While more study is needed to conclusively prove the value of this herb in relieving tinnitus symptoms, it may be worth a try. Ginkgo is easy to obtain at most any health food store, is safe to use and inexpensive.

Yoga Breathing Exercises

As we have already established in this book, yoga is often useful in stress reduction. Several specific yoga breathing techniques (that help clear the inner ear and sinus cavities) may be useful for tinnitus sufferers.

Here is how to do them:

◊ Sit comfortably with your lower back well supported, your head upright and your shoulders back.

◊ Inhale normally through both nostrils. Hold one nostril closed and exhale through the other open nostril.

◊ Inhale again through both nostrils. Hold the other nostril closed and exhale through the open nostril.

◊ Repeat the second and third steps, alternating breathing from one nostril to the other. Do this two to three times a day for about five minutes each session. It should take about two minutes to "pop" each ear, an act that helps promote cleansing of the ears.

For a more vigorous technique, inhale and exhale one nostril at a time simply by alternately holding one nostril closed. If your nasal passages are blocked, you may be able to unclog them by inhaling through your mouth and gently exhaling through the less-blocked nostril until it clears, then repeating for the other side.

Relief from Sounds

Dr. Deepak Chopra of Del Mar, California, is a nationally prominent medical doctor who subscribes to alternative treatments to treat health problems. In his audio presentation *Magical Mind, Magical Body*, Dr. Chopra recommends uttering the letter "n" for as long as comfortably possible.

To practice this exercise, sit in a comfortable position and simply utter "n"—almost as if you were humming "nnnnnnnnn." Try this three times a day, for several minutes each session. Many people have reported good results using Chopra's exercise.

Morning Tinnitus— Some Helpful Suggestions

Some tinnitus sufferers experience a significant increase in tinnitus in the morning, a condition sometimes called "morning roar." Some people achieve relief from morning roar by sleeping with their head slightly elevated through the use of extra pillows. The specific reason why this alleviates symptoms in some people has not been scientifically established. However, it's believed that elevating the head during sleep may help relieve congestion of blood in the ear canal.

In other cases, morning roar may be caused by a drop in blood-sugar levels while sleeping. Many people report relief by consuming sugar first thing in the morning. This is normally accomplished by putting a tablespoon of sugar in your favorite morning beverage or drinking a small glass of warm water with a tablespoon of sugar. Others get good results from a glass of fresh orange juice.

CHAPTER 11

How Hearing Works

To fully understand the various things that can go wrong with our hearing—including the possible development of tinnitus—it's useful to understand how human hearing works.

Hearing—which can be roughly defined as the receiving and the interpretation of sounds—is an extremely complex process, involving many different aspects. Although the ears are generally viewed as the organs of hearing, the correct recognition of sounds also requires the proper functioning of the auditory pathway—a series of stages through which nerve impulses are eventually transmitted to the brain.

Let us start by looking at the ear, which consists of three main parts:

157

1. The outer ear (also known as the *external ear*). This consists not only of what is commonly called the ear (the flap of skin and cartilage on the side of the head), but also includes the tube that leads from the ear to the eardrum;

2. The middle ear (also known as the *tympanum* or the *tympanic cavity*) is an irregularly shaped air-filled cavity located beyond the eardrum where the vibrations received by the eardrum are transmitted via a series of small bones to the oval window which lies at the start of the inner ear.

3. The inner ear (also known as the internal ear or sometimes referred to as the *labyrinth*). This part of the ear is made up of a convoluted system of cavities and ducts, most of which are concerned with maintaining balance, but it also contains a large central cavity (the *cochlea*) where the received sound impulses are processed and transformed into signals that stimulate the nerves of hearing.

Let us look at these various parts in greater detail.

The Outer Ear

There are two parts to the outer ear: the *auricle* or *pinna* (that is the visible part which lies outside the head); and the external *auditory meatus*, a tube that leads through the temporal bone of the skull to the eardrum.

The auricle serves but little (if any) auditory purpose in man as it's too small to make a great contribution to the efficiency of the collection of sound.

Inside the auricle lies a hollow (called the *concha*) and it is in the deepest part of this that the external auditory meatus begins. This meatus is usually about an inch long and slightly curved in shape, with approximately the first third of it cartilaginous and the remaining two thirds bony.

The external auditory meatus is lined throughout by skin, which contains both sebaceous and ceruminous glands, the latter believed to be sweat glands that are modified so that instead of secreting sweat they produce *cerumen,* the medical name for ear wax. An excessive production and/or accumulation of ear wax can be responsible for both deafness and tinnitus, something that is dealt with in greater detail in Chapter 4.

The Middle Ear

At the innermost end of the outer ear's external auditory canal lies the eardrum, a membrane made of skin and very thin collagen fibers that, unless damaged, completely seals off the outer ear from the middle ear. A muscle (the tensor timpani) that runs from the ear drum to the wall of the middle ear keeps the ear drum under tension, making it responsive to sound waves.

A chain of very small bones (called the *auditory ossicles*) are located in the middle ear and their job is to transmit and magnify the vibrations perceived by the ear drum to the oval window which lies at the opposite end of the middle ear. There are three ossicles, the first two acting as levers upon the next one in the chain and the last one acting directly upon the opening to the inner ear:

⬥ The first ossicle is the hammer (the *malleus*). It is attached to the upper part of the ear drum and therefore responds to vibrations induced there by sound waves, transmitting and amplifying these to the next ossicle.

⬥ In the middle of the chain is the anvil (the *incus*). This receives vibrations from the hammer, and amplifies these once more, before transmitting them further along the line.

⬥ Last in the chain is the stirrup (the *stapes*), its non medical name stemming from its shape which resembles a stirrup. The innermost end of the stirrup lies directly upon the oval window, the small opening in the skull that marks the entrance to the inner ear. The stirrup receives vibrations from the anvil and amplifies these as it transmits them to the oval window.

As you can see, the ossicles provide three separate stages at which the sound vibrations are magnified, the amount of amplification becoming greater and greater as the vibrations proceed along the chain.

However, apart from that produced by the lever effect of the ossicles, further amplification also takes place within the middle ear because vibrations captured by the ear drum—which has a relatively large surface (averaging 85 square millimeters) are eventually received by the oval window whose average surface is only 3.2 square millimeters. This difference in surface areas creates amplification because when the same amount of force is applied to a smaller surface, its intensity is increased.

One way of understanding this effect is by thinking of a given amount of rain falling. If all the rain is spread over a large surface—like a lawn—then each square foot of it will only receive a small amount. However, should the same quantity of rain be concentrated within a single square foot that area would indeed be subjected to a veritable deluge.

The two amplification processes in the middle ear—the lever action of the ossicles plus that resulting from the different sizes of the surfaces of the ear drum and oval window—combine to bring about a massive total amount of amplification, the vibrations reaching the inner ear being between 20 and 25 times more powerful than they were when originally received by the ear drum. Because the effect of this magnification can in fact become too intense when the sound level is extremely high, there is also a mechanism through which it can be automatically damped down and this consists of a muscle (the *stampede* muscle) that reduces the build up of oscillations in the ossicles by pulling the stirrup somewhat away from the oval window. Unfortunately, this damping down effect depends on reflex action and this reacts too slowly to allow people to avoid the damage that may be caused by very sudden and extremely loud noises, such as gunfire.

Other Aspects of the Middle Ear

As has been noted briefly, the middle ear (like the outer ear) is an air-filled cavity. It is vital that the air pressure within both the inner and the outer ears be the same. Should the pressures not be equal, the ear drum would become artificially distended inward or outward, depending upon whether the air pressure in the middle ear was higher of lower than that created by atmospheric pressure in the outer ear. This equalization of pressure is achieved though very narrow conduits (the *Eustachian tubes*). Most of the time, the Eustachian tubes are closed. But they open— in response to involuntary muscular action— when you swallow or yawn. If the pressure in the middle ear is not identical with atmospheric pressure, then either more air will be admitted to or some will be released from the middle ear through these tubes.

Of course, it would seem that the whole problem of matching the air pressure in the middle ear to that of atmospheric pressure would never have arisen had Mother Nature chosen to design the Eustachian tubes so that they were permanently open. There is, however, a very good reason why the tubes are closed most of the time as this reduces the risk of infection affecting the middle ear. This natural fail-safe mechanism can nevertheless be defeated when you blow your nose too violently as this can drive infected material through the Eustachian tubes into the middle ear, possibly resulting in earache or temporarily diminished hearing.

It also needs to be noted that the middle ear provides another important function as it transforms the sound vibrations captured by the ear drum— which, of course, are vibrations occurring in the air—into vibrations which are better suited for being transmitted in fluid, the inner ear lying at the other side of the oval window being a fluid filled cavity. Fluid offers a different kind of resistance to the transmission of vibrations than air and this is also one of the reasons why the signals received by the ear drum have to be amplified before they reach the inner ear.

The Inner Ear

On the other side of the oval window lies the inner ear. It is filled with a special fluid called *perilymph* and contains a number of cavities, most of which are concerned with balance, but also one (the *cochlea*) where sound vibrations are transformed into impulses which can travel along the nerves to the brain. The cochlea is a tube within which lie three more tubes. Overall the cochlea is spiral-shaped, looking rather like a snail's shell. The widest part of the cochlea lies near and just below the oval window. Just below, the cochlea is also linked to another window (the *round window*) that lies between the middle and the inner ear.

The three tubes within the cochlea are:

1. The *scalai vestibuli,* also called the *vestibular canal.* This is open to the perilymph of the inner ear.

2. The *scala tympany,* also called the *tympanic canal.* This tube also contains peri-

lymph and links to the round window. The scala vestibuli and the scala tympany are in fact connected by a very small opening (the *helicotrema*) at the very end of the cochlea, but the size of this opening is so minute that it greatly restricts the amount of perilymph that can flow through it.

3. Sandwiched between these two tubes is the third one, the *cochlear duct* (also called the *scala media*), which is filled with a different fluid (*endolymph*) and contains the *organ of Corti* (also known as the *spiral organ*), a very complex structure that converts sound signals into nerve impulses that are transmitted via the cochlear nerve to the brain.

The cochlea marks an important stage in the process of hearing because it is here that sounds that hitherto had been vibrations, transmitted through the air, via resonating bones or membranes, or through fluid, are metamorphosed into nerve impulses that can be sent to and recognized by the brain. Broadly speaking, this is how the sounds are changed from one form into the other:

◇ Vibrations resulting from the action of the stapes on the oval window are transmitted via the perilymph to the scala vestibuli of the cochlea.

◊ The vibrations affect the pressure in the both the scala vestibuli and the scala tim- pani. Naturally, these changes in pressure also affect the cochlear duct as it lies be- tween the other two scalas.

◊ As already mentioned, within the co- chlear duct is the organ of Corti and this, in part, consists of a continuous mem- brane (the *basilar membrane*) within which are embedded some 30,000 sen- sory cells from which protrude very thin hairs. The upper ends of these hairs are embedded in another membrane, the *tec- torial membrane*.

◊ As the cochlear duct becomes distorted in response to altering pressures in the surrounding scalas, this distortion also affects the tectorial membrane, causing it to exert a tugging action on the hair cells. The stimulus created by this pull- ing action then triggers the hair cells into setting off nervous impulses which are then transmitted by nerve fibers to even- tually reach the brain.

Maintaining Balance

The inner ear also contains other cavities whose correct functioning, although not directly con-

166

nected with hearing, can also become affected when there is inner ear infection. In certain instances, hearing problems will also be accompanied by disturbances in the sense of balance. This combination of symptoms, of course, is a pointer strongly suggesting that the origin of disorder is likely to be somewhere in the inner ear. For that reason, it's worth taking a brief look at these other organs, which include:

⬧ Three semicircular canals—one of which lies more or less horizontally and two of which are placed vertically with their planes at 90 degrees to each other. These three structures can be said to represent two adjoining sides and the floor a cube. Each of these canals is about 15mm long and lies within ducts in the bone of the skull. At the end of each canal lies a somewhat wider area (the *ampulla*) that contains sensory cells which detect movements in the fluid within the canals and then translate this information into nervous impulses.

⬧ The *utriculus* (also called the *utricle*)—an endolymph-filled membranous sac that contains a sensory macula that lies more or less horizontally and whose hairs respond to gravity and translate this data into nervous impulses that are sent to the brain, providing the latter with information about how the head is currently positioned.

◊ The *sacculus* (also known as the *saccule*)—is similar to but much smaller than the utriculus. It also contains a sensory macula, but one that is positioned more or less vertically and that responds to gravity and provides the brain with information about the position of the head. There is, however, some doubt about the exact role of the sacculus in humans, some experts believing that it may not play a large role in controlling balance, but may instead be partly involved in hearing, especially in the recognition of sounds of very low frequencies.

This is how these five separate, but cross-linked, organs work in harmony to control both body balance and posture:

◊ The three semicircular canals—acting together like a trio of building floors—provide the brain with the information it needs to maintain the body's overall balance, this being achieved through setting off reflex actions in various muscles to place the body in the currently desired position.

◊ On the other hand, the utriculus—aided to some extent by the sacculus—provides the brain with the information it needs to maintain posture.

Naturally, the brain also receives information about balance and posture from other sources, notably from the eyes and feedback from various muscles and all of this additional data is amalgamated with that which is coming from the inner ear cavities. Dizziness, poor balance, deficient coordination are all problems that can arise when there is a discord between the information coming from different sources, as can happen through disease or malfunctioning of one or more of the organs involved or when seemingly conflicting information is received, such as during a ride on a helter-skelter.

In a Nutshell

To sum up the above, this is what happens in the ear during the process of hearing:

1. The sound impulses—transmitted in the air as vibrations—are received by the outer ear, the auricle serving as a not too efficient funnel that helps direct the vibrations into the external auditory meatus.

2. At the end of the external auditory meatus lies the ear drum and the sound impulses cause this membrane to vibrate.

3. On the inner side of the ear drum are the ossicles which together act as chain

along which the vibrations are amplified before being delivered to the oval window that separates the middle ear from the inner ear.

4. In the inner ear, the vibrations transmitted to the oval window from the ossicles are then transmitted via a fluid to the cochlea where the vibrations are transformed into nerve impulses.

The Vestibulocochlear Nerve

The sensory impulses generated in the inner ear are carried to the brain along the *Vestibulocochlear nerve.* This is the eighth of 12 pairs of cranial nerves and is also known as the *auditory nerve* or *acoustic nerve,* and in medical texts is often indicated by the Roman numeral "VIII."

The vestibulocochlear nerve has two branches:

1. The *cochlear nerve* is the nerve of hearing as it carries the impulses originating in the cochlea.

2. The *vestibular nerve* carries the impulses from the semicircular canals, utricles and saccules—information about balance, posture, and movement.

The auditory pathways connecting the ears to the brain also have a number of "stations" along the way where nervous impulses are further processed. There are also interconnections between various corresponding stations in the left and the right pathways which allow for the comparison of information collected by the left and right ear, this comparison being part of the process through which the brain determines from which direction particular sound came.

What Can Go Wrong

Even from this simplified description of the hearing process, it's obvious that difficulties in hearing may be caused by a problem anywhere along it line of transmission. Things that can go wrong and impair hearing, either temporarily or permanently, include:

◊ In the outer ear, the channel may become obstructed by wax, this physical obstruction stopping sound waves from reaching the ear drum.

◊ The ear drum can be damaged and therefore become unable to correctly receive vibrations.

◊ Ossicles can fail to work properly, so reducing the degree of amplification their lever actions normally produce.

◊ Various diseases (discussed in Chapter 4) can interfere with or interrupt the transmission of sound vibrations.

◊ Additionally, any of the three parts of the ear can become infected and inflamed, a condition called *otitis,* of which there are three main forms:

1. *Otitis externa* describes inflammation of the outer ear. This occurs frequently in swimmers and is also known as *swimmer's ear.*

2. *Otitis media* is inflammation occurring in the middle ear and resulting from bacterial or viral infection. Treatment usually consists of antibiotics. Similar to this is *secretory otitis media*—also known as *glue ear*—a condition marked by the chronic accumulation of fluid in the middle ear and which often treated by a relatively minor procedure during which a double-cuffed tube, called a grommet, is inserted in the ear drum to allow excess fluid to drain from the middle ear. Common symptoms of middle ear infection include moderate to severe pain and a high fever.

3. *Otitis interna* (also called *labyrinthitis*) refers to inflammation of the middle ear.

Common symptoms include dizziness, an impaired sense of balance, and vomiting.

Naturally, any kind of ear infection needs prompt professional attention as without it the hearing may become permanently impaired.

Summing Things Up

The process of hearing is a very intricate one and metamorphosing air vibrations created by sound into nervous impulses the brain can interpret involves several quite separate stages, all of which need to be functioning properly to provide normal hearing.

CHAPTER 12

Where to Get More Information—

U.S. Resources

American Tinnitus Association
1618 Southwest 1st Ave., Portland, OR 97201
PO Box 5, Portland, OR 97207-0005
Tel: 503-248-9985 Toll Free: 800-634-8978
Fax: 503-248-0024
Website: www.ata.org
E-mail: tinnitus@ata.org

The American Tinnitus Association (ATA) is a national organization of self-help groups devoted to providing support for tinnitus sufferers. The

ATA offers referrals to professional health care providers in your area who specialize in treating tinnitus. The ATA also publishes a quarterly newsletter and offers a wide array of information on tinnitus.

National Health Information Center
Tel:1-800-336-4797
Website: www.Health.Gov/NHIC

The NHIC is a free federal government service that provides information, answers questions and makes referrals on health-related topics.

American Academy of Otolaryngology
1 Prince St, Alexandria, VA 22314
Tel: 703-836-444
Fax: 703-683-5100
Website: www.entnet.org

The Academy represents more than 10,000 otolaryngologists who diagnose and treat disorders of the ears, nose, throat, and related structures of the head and neck. The AAO-HNS Foundation works to advance the art, science and ethical practice of otolaryngology (head and neck surgery) through education, research and lifelong learning.

American Academy of Audiology
11730 Plaza America Dr, # 300, Reston,
VA 20190

Tel: 703-790-8466 Toll free: 800-AAA-2336
Fax: 703-790-8631
Website: www.audiology.org
Email: info@audiology.org

The AAA website offers the latest industry news for professionals and consumers, continuing education features as well as a search engine for audiologists within the United States and abroad.

Sight & Hearing Association
674 Transfer Rd, St Paul, MN 55114-1402
Tel: 651-645-2546 Toll free: 800-992-0424
Fax: 651-645-2742
Website: www.Sightandhearing.com
Email: mail@sightandhearing.org

This non-profit organization works to prevent the needless loss of vision and hearing through the development of effective screening, education and research programs. Besides general information on hearing-related matters, the sight includes a quick hearing test.

Tinnitus Treatment and Research Centers—California Tinnitus Center
4747 Mission Blvd., #6, San Diego, CA 92109
Tel: 858-270-4575
Website: www.californiatinnitus.com
Email: dr.bob@cox.net

Promotes tinnitus retraining therapy (also known as habituation therapy) based on the theory that any person can habituate to acoustic or acoustic-like sensations in their environment.

House Ear Institute
2100 W. 3rd St, Los Angeles, CA 90057
Tel: 213-483-9930
TDD: 213-483-5706
Website: www.hei.org/welcome.htm

Massachusetts Eye and Ear Infirmary
243 Charles St, Boston, MA 02114-3096
Tel: 617-573-5520
Fax: 617-573-3444
Website: www.meei.harvard.edu
Email: ral@epl.harvard.edu

Martha Entenmann Tinnitus Research Center
118-35 Queens Blvd, # 1430, Forest Hills, NY 11375
Tel. 718- 773-8888
Fax: 718-465-3669
Website: www.tinnituscenter.com

Southeastern Comprehensive Tinnitus Clinic
980 Johnson Ferry Rd, N.E. #760, Atlanta, GA 30342
Tel: 404-531-3979
Website: www.mindspring.com/~nagler

The Tinnitus Clinic, Oregon Hearing Research Center, Oregon Health Sciences University

3181 SW Sam Jackson Park Rd., Portland, OR 97201

Tel: 503-494-7954

Website: www.ohsu.edu/ohrc/tinnitusclinic/tusclinic/

University of Maryland Tinnitus and Hyperacusis Center

419 W. Redwood Center

Baltimore, MD 21201

Tel: 410-328-1279

Website: www.tinnitus-hyperacusis.com

Acupuncture

International College of Acupuncture & Electro-Therapeutics

800 Riverside Dr. (8-I), New York, NY 10032

Tel: 212-781-6262

Fax: 212-923-2279

Website: www.icaet.org

This nonprofit education organization, chartered by the University of the State of New York, promotes research and teaching of safe and effective acupuncture and related treatments including herbal medicine. It works to combine the best of Western and Oriental medicine through international cooperation and shares its findings with the public.

HealthWorld Online, Inc.
4049 Lyceum Ave, Los Angeles, CA 90066
Website: www.healthy.net
Email: info@healthy.net

HealthWorld Online offers vast resources in nutrition, fitness, self-care and mind/body approaches to maintaining high-level health. This 24-hour health resource center offers a virtual "health village" where you can access information, products and services to create your wellness-based lifestyle.

Journal of Alternative and Complementary Medicine
2 Madison Ave, Larchmont, NY 10538
Tel: 914-834-3100 Toll free: 800-654-3237
Fax: 914-834-3688
Website: www.liebertpub.com
Email: info@liebertpub.com

The journal includes observational and analytical reports on treatments outside the realm of allopathic medicine which are gaining interest and warrant research to assess their therapeutic value. This organization publishes a monthly newsletter devoted to alternative and complementary medicine.

National Association for Holistic Aromatherapy (NAHA)

4509 Interlake Ave. N., # 233
Seattle, WA 98103-6773
Tel: 888-ASK-NAHA or 206-547-2164
Fax: 206-547-2680
Website: www.naha.org
Email: info@naha.org

This group publishes a quarterly "Aromatherapy Journal." More than 60 aromatic substances exhibit healing properties. When applied to the skin, these substances can aid healing. When inhaled, proponents believe they trigger a reaction in the brain which can achieve therapeutic effects.

National Center for Complementary and Alternative Medicine

P.O. Box 7923
Gaithersburg, MD 20898
Toll Free: 888-644-6226
Website: www.nccam.nih.gov
Email: info@nccam.nih.gov

NCCAM is one of the 27 institutes and centers that make up the National Institutes of Health (NIH). Its mission is to support research on complementary and alternative medicine (CAM), to train researchers in CAM, and to disseminate information on the effectiveness of CAM modalities.

Biofeedback

Association for Applied Psycho-physiology & Biofeedback (AAPB)
10200 West 44th Ave, Suite 304, Wheat
Ridge, CO 80033-2840
Tel: 303-422-8436
Fax: 303-422-8894
Website: www.aapb.org
Email: aapb@resourcenter.com

AAPB pursues continuing study in biofeedback—
a technique in which people are taught to improve their health and performance by using signals from their own bodies. The organization
embraces more than 2,000 members in most
states. It can provide referrals to qualified professionals in your area.

Chelation Therapy

The American College for Advancement in Medicine
23121 Verdugo Dr, #204, Laguna Hills, CA
92653
Tel: 800-LEAD-OUT
Fax: 949-455-9679
Website: www.acam.org
Email: info@acam.org

This nonprofit medical society is dedicated to educating physicians and other health-care profession-

als on the latest findings and emerging procedures in preventive/nutritional medicine including chelation. Free information on chelation therapy (explaining the health benefits, cost and insurance coverage) is available upon request. Chelation therapy was developed to remove heavy metals (like lead and mercury) from the body. In a more controversial application, chelation is sometimes used as a means for clearing other kinds of deposits from the arteries, removing obstructions and improving blood circulation.

Otolaryngology

American Academy of Otolaryngology
One Prince Street, Alexandria, VA 22314-3357
Tel: 703-836-4444
Website: www.entnet.org

Provides a variety of free information on topics associated with the ears, nose and throat and related structures of the head and neck. Some of the publications available include material on earwax, TMJ and tinnitus.

Food Allergies

Allergy Alert
P.O. Box 31065, Seattle, WA 98103

Tel: 206-547-1814
Fax: 206-547-7696
Website: www.arxc.com/rockwell/letter.htm

Issues a self-help newsletter with articles on the latest food-allergy research, cooking tips and proper diet information.

Healing Centers

Body Mind Spirit Directory
Website: www.BodyMindSpiritDirectory.org
Email: source@one.net

An online list of practitioners and products that are natural, holistic, metaphysical, spiritual or healing related. Use this national directory to find links to centers and associations providing holistic health, healing, spirituality and metaphysical services.

Hearing Problems

Self Help for Hard of Hearing People (SHHH)
7910 Woodmont Ave, # 1200
Bethesda, Maryland 20814
Tel: 301-657-2248 TTY: 301-657-2249
Fax: 301-913-9413
Website: www.shhh.org

Email: national@shhh.org

SHHH provides self-help tools to people with hearing loss; educates the general population about the special needs of people who are hard of hearing; and promotes understanding of the nature, causes, complications and remedies of hearing loss.

National Association for Hearing and Speech Action (NHSA)

10801 Rockville Pike, Rockville, MD 20852
Tel: 800-638-8255

This association is an information and resource center for the American Speech/Language/Hearing Association. A number of helpful publications are available and the NHSA offers referrals to audiologists and speech and language therapists.

Hearing Education and Awareness for Rockers (H.E.A.R.)

PO Box 460847, San Francisco, CA 94146
Tel: 415-773-9590
Website: Hearnet.com
Email: hear@hearnet.com

This grassroots organization was started by Kathy Peck and physician Flash Gordon in San Francisco. Peck, a former base player for a band called The Contractions, was affected by tinnitus and hearing loss after repeated exposure to excessive noise. H.E.A.R. is now recognized around the world for its efforts in educating the public on the dangers of excessive noise and providing adequate hearing protection for musicians and music fans.

Herbalism

American Botanical Council (ABC)
6200 Manor Rd, Austin, TX 78723
Tel: 512- 926-4900
Fax: 512- 926-2345
Website: herbalgram.org
Email: abc@herbalgram.org

This nonprofit council conducts research and disseminates information on the safe and effective use of medicinal plants. It publishes a quarterly newsletter.

American Herbal Products Association (AHPA)
8484 Georgia Ave., #370, Silver Spring, MD 20910
Tel: 301-588-1171
Fax: 301-588-1174
Website: www.ahpa.org
Email: ahpa@ahpa.org

AHPA promotes the responsible commerce of products which contain herbs used to enhance health and quality of life. The group's Botanical Safety Handbook contains information (in an easy-to-use classification system) on more than 600 commonly sold herbs.

Medical Herbalism

Website: www.medherb.com

This site provides links to medical information and other resources relevant to medicinal herbs or herbalism practiced in a clinical setting. Includes book reviews, newsletters, history, nutrition, reference sources and data on adverse effects.

Homeopathy

National Center for Homeopathy (NCH)
801 North Fairfax St., #306, Alexandria, VA 22314
Tel: 877-624-0613 or 703-548-7790
Fax: 703-548-7792
Website: www.homeopathic.org
Email: info@homeopathic.org

A nonprofit membership organization dedicated to making homeopathy accessible to the general public. Its mission is to promote good health through homeopathy. The NCH magazine Homeopathy Today contains up-to-date news, tips, short articles and a calendar of events and the group's library contains one of the largest collections of homeopathic literature in the U.S.

Hypnosis

Academy of Scientific Hypnotherapy
P.O. Box 12041
San Diego, CA 92112-3041
Tel: 619-427-6225
Fax: 619-427-5650

The academy acts as a clearinghouse for information and makes referrals to local hypnotherapists.

The National Society of Hypnotherapists
1833 W. Charleston Blvd, Las Vegas, NV
    89102.
Tel: 702-384-4420.
Website: www.wel.net/katherine/2/nsh.html
Email: LKKeck@aol.com

Publishes a monthly newsletter on new developments in hypnotherapy and makes referrals to qualified hypnotherapists in your area.

Naturopathy

The American Association of Naturopathic Physicians (AANP)
3201 New Mexico Ave, NW # 350, Washington DC 20016
Tel: 866-538-2267 or 202-895-1392
Fax: 202-274-1992
Website: www.naturopathic.org

Email: member.services@Naturopathic.org

In addition to the basic medical sciences and conventional diagnostics, naturopathic practitioners provide services in therapeutic nutrition, botanical medicine, homeopathy, natural childbirth, classical Chinese medicine, hydrotherapy, naturopathic manipulative therapy, pharmacology and minor surgery. Naturopathic medicine concentrates on whole-patient wellness and attempts to find the underlying cause of the patient's condition rather than focusing solely on symptomatic treatment.

Nutrition and Diet

Certification Board for Nutrition Specialists (CBNS)
300 S. Duncan Ave., #225, Clearwater, FL 33755
Tel: 727-446-6086
Fax: 727-446-6202
Website: www.cert-nutrition.org
E-mail: Office@cert-nutrition.org

This board helps establish standards and certifies those who are able to pass an examination. The board can provide a list of qualified professional nutritionists in your area. Its website also provides links to the American College of Nutrition and the college's bimonthly publication, Journal of the American College of Nutrition.

Self-Help Groups

American Self-Help Clearing House
50 Morris Avenue
Denville, NJ 07834
Website: www.mentalhelp.net/selfhelp

This organization provides assistance in finding national and local self-help groups. It also publishes a nationwide directory of self-help groups.

Alt.support.tinnitus

The Usenet newsgroup alt.support.tinnitus is an Internet discussion forum where you can talk and exchange advice with other tinnitus sufferers. Please note, however, that this newsgroup is un-censored and unmoderated, so you never know what you are going to find there.

CHAPTER 13

Where to Get More Information—

International Resources

AUSTRALIA

Australian Tinnitus Association
2 Leichhardt St, Darlinghurst NSW 2010
PO Box 660, Woollahra NSW 1350, Australia
Tel: 011- 61- 02 8382 3331
Fax: 011-61-02 8382 3333
Website: tinnitus.asn.au
Email: info@tinnitus.asn.au

Established in 1984 and is supported by the South
Eastern Sydney Area Health Service, ATA's mis-

sion is to provide information, support and counseling to tinnitus sufferers and preventative education to the wider community. The website offers links to tinnitus associations and self-help groups in other Australian states and features a kids' corner.

CANADA

Tinnitus Association of Canada (TAC)
23 Ellis Park Rd, Toronto, ON M6S 2V4
    Canada
Tel: 416-762-1490
Website: www.kadis.com/ta/tinnitus.htm

Operated on a voluntary basis by people who suffer from tinnitus, this nonprofit organization shares practical information on ways to reduce the distress of chronic head and ear noises. TAC is the only Canadian charity with English-language information on the problem of tinnitus.

GREAT BRITAIN

British Tinnitus Association (BTA)
Ground Floor, Unit 5, Acorn Business Park, Woodseats Close, Sheffield, S8 0TB, England
Tel: 0-800-018-0527 or 0845 4500 321
    (within the UK); 44-0-114-250-9922
    outside the UK
Fax: 011-44-258-2279

Website: www.tinnitus.org.uk
Email: info@tinnitus.org.uk
The only national British charity exclusively devoted to tinnitus, the British Tinnitus Association defines its primary mission as "the relief and ultimate cure of permanent head noises." Its current activities include:

⬦ Supporting (and helping to establish) local self-help groups.

⬦ Providing assistance for research into tinnitus.

⬦ Seeking greater public recognition of the disorder.

⬦ Publishing a quarterly journal called Quiet that provides advice on the relief of tinnitus and also reports on the latest clinical and scientific research.

⬦ Playing a leading role in the international exchange of information between tinnitus associations in many countries.

The Royal National Institute for Deaf People (RNID)
19-23 Featherstone St, London EC1Y 8SL, England
Tel: 011-44-808-808-0123
Text phone: 011-44-808-808-9000

Fax: 011-44-020-7296-8199
Website: www.rnid.org.uk
E-mail: informationline@rnid.org.uk

RNID is the largest voluntary organization in Britain representing the needs of deaf, deafened, hard of hearing, and deaf and blind people. Group aims include increasing public awareness and understanding of deafness and deaf people, and campaigning to remove prejudice and discrimination by raising issues in the Press and in Parliament.

The institute also provides a wide range of quality services for deaf people and the professionals who work with them, including information, residential care, communications support, training, specialist telephone services and various assisting devices.

USEFUL INTERNATIONAL WEBSITES

http://www.eskimo.com/~carol/T.html
The Tinnitus Online Community includes chat rooms, news groups, message boards and e-mail updates for people with tinnitus.

http://www.haruteq.com/tin-01.htm
This website, which appears to have been constructed by German Bart Veerman, offers useful links to doctors, support groups and newsgroups worldwide.

www.britishservices.co.uk/altmed.htm
is an online source for alternative medical groups in Britain.

www.mca.gov.uk/home.htm
is the website of the British Medicines Control Agency.

For more general information, surf the following sites:

www.bixby.org/faq/tinnitus.html

**www.hearusa.com/tinnitus/
tinnitus_home.html**

www.tinnitusanswerboard.com

RESEARCH

At the time of publication, a number of interesting research studies were being carried out on tinnitus. Mentioning them in this book doesn't mean the research will lead to results of any significance and this is by no means an exhaustive list of the research being carried out on this subject today.

Researchers at Tubingen University in Germany are currently conducting a study based on the premise that the noise that some patients hear when suffering from tinnitus could be some sort of phantom auditory perception similar to phantom pain. Led by Christian Gerloff, the researchers are working on jamming some of the brain's activity that could be leading to the illusion of noise. A test on 14 patients, in which a pulsed magnetic field was directed to the areas of the brain associated with auditory systems, brought mixed results, with eight patients reporting a period of silence, five reporting no change and one reporting worsening of the tinnitus.

Studies at the University of Western Australia are looking at the neural noise measured at the round window in the middle ear, which may help in diagnosing the location of tinnitus generators. These researchers are also assessing the electrical voltage changes in the ear with a view to regulating electrical charges to lessen tinnitus.

Clinicians at Curtin University of Technology in Perth, Australia are comparing and contrasting different combinations of tinnitus management and treatment including desensitization music, masking music, masking noise and counseling. They report that total masking with music and intermittent music reduces awareness and improves relaxation.

Boston-based doctors Levine, Abel and Cheng (and the Massachusetts Eye and Ear Infirmary, Massachusetts General Hospital, Harvard Medical School, Harvard Dental School and the Massachusetts Institute of Technology) are compiling a growing body of evidence that links clinical tinnitus to the somatosensory system. In their tests, about 80% of non-clinical subjects who had ongoing tinnitus could adjust their tinnitus with forceful contractions of their heads and necks. Almost 60% of those with no tinnitus at the time of testing could elicit tinnitus-like sounds with head and neck contractions.

Index

NOTES

NOTES

NOTES

NOTES

NOTES

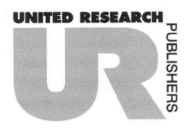

UNITED RESEARCH PUBLISHERS

United Research Publishers publishes books and videos on Health & Relief, Diet & Fitness, and Better Living & Self-Improvement topics. All of our publications are dedicated to improving the quality of day-to-day living.

Health & Relief Books and Videos
The Complete Handbook of Health Tips
The Fibromyalgia Relief Handbook
The Gout Relief Handbook
The Irritable Bowel Syndrome and Gastro-Intestinal Solutions Handbook
The Macular Degeneration Handbook
The Panic Attack, Anxiety & Phobia Solutions Handbook
The Prostate Handbook—What Every Man Over 40 Needs to Know About His Prostate
The Psoriasis Handbook - A Self-Help Guide
The Rosacea Handbook - A Self-Help Guide
The Sciatica Relief Handbook
The Sinus Handbook: A Self-Help Guide
Stopping Restless Leg Syndrome
Tinnitus: The Complete Self-Help Guide
Impotence (Video)
Irritable Bowel Syndrome (Video)
The Prostate (Video)

Diet & Fitness Books and Videos
Calorie Neutralizing Foods (Book)
3 Simple Steps to Flatten Your Belly (Book)
7-Minute Abdominal Workout (Video)
Calorie Combining for Weight Loss (Video)

Better Living & Self-Improvement Books
Living Easy in Mexico
*Paradise Found: How to Live in North America
     for Under $500/Month*
Effortless Internet Handbook
Write Perfect Letters for Any Occasion
*Common Embarrassing Mistakes in English
     and How to Correct Them*
Complete Handbook of US Government Benefits
50 Secrets to Meet People & Make Friends
Complete Books of Gardening Tips
*How You Can Achieve Financial Independence
     in Mail Order*

For more information contact us using any of the following means:

United Research Publishers
PO Box 232344
Encinitas, CA 92023
Phone: 760-930-8937
Fax: 760-930-4291
Email: contactus@urpublishers.com
Web: www.urpublishers.com